RESUSCITATION
CONTROVERSIAL ASPECTS

RESUSCITATION
CONTROVERSIAL ASPECTS

AN INTERNATIONAL SYMPOSIUM

HELD AT THE FIRST EUROPEAN CONGRESS OF ANAESTHESIOLOGY
OF THE
WORLD FEDERATION OF SOCIETIES OF ANAESTHESIOLOGISTS

VIENNA / AUSTRIA, SEPTEMBER 5, 1962

CHAIRMAN AND EDITOR

PETER SAFAR, M. D.
PITTSBURGH, U. S. A.

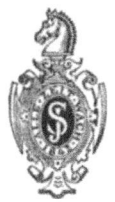

Springer-Verlag Berlin Heidelberg GmbH 1963

© by Springer-Verlag Berlin Heidelberg 1963
Originally published by Springer-Verlag OHG Berlin . Göttinge . Heidelberg in 1963

Library of Congress Catalog Card Number 63-18770

ISBN 978-3-540-03050-8   ISBN 978-3-642-88100-8 (eBook)
DOI 10.1007/978-3-642-88100-8

Printed by Konrad Triltsch, Graphischer Großbetrieb, Würzburg

Preface

The First European Congress of Anesthesiology in Vienna, Austria in September, 1962 presented 19 Symposium discussions, each lasting approximately 3 hours. Unlike most of these panels, the one on Resuscitation was a free discussion on controversial topics, without presentation of formal papers.

In spite of the spontaneity of the unrehearsed questions and answers, the participants felt that an edited version of this Symposium should be published. The reasons for publication included the international character of the group of participants and the recent general interest in respiratory and circulatory resuscitation.

A presentation of accepted resuscitation techniques was omitted, because of lack of time and because the Symposium was held primarily for trained anesthesiologists, most of whom have first-hand experience with resuscitation and should be familiar with the accepted modern methods. Only controversial topics, which seemed to be of interest to those with personal experience in the application and the research of resuscitation, were included.

For clarity, parts of the taped discussion had to be re-worded in the following written presentation. This was possible without changing the meaning of the speakers' statements. Often the Chairman of an informal panel runs out of time in his attempt to cover all the questions he intended to ask the participants. Since this Symposium was no exception in this respect, a few topics and the Summary, which could not be presented at the meeting because of lack of time, have been added in this written version. The additional answers and pertinent literature references were collected by the Chairman through correspondence.

The following pages are not to be considered a teaching text. They merely represent conclusions concerning some basic concepts of resuscitation techniques drawn at this time by a few specialists. In this continuously changing field we hope that the following discussion will stimulate interest in the critical appraisal of clinical resuscitation attempts and in more controlled investigations.

Pittsburgh (U.S.A.)   PETER SAFAR

Contents

Participants

LEROY C. HARRIS, JR. . . . Department of Anesthesiology,
University of Pittsburgh,
Pittsburgh (U.S.A.)

MARTIN HOLMDAHL . . . Department of Anaesthesiology,
University of Uppsala,
Uppsala (Sweden)

ERNEST KERN . . . . Department of Anaesthesiology,
University of Paris,
Paris (France)

HUGO KESZLER . . . . Institute for Clinical and Experimental Surgery,
University of Prague,
Prague (ČSR)

RUDOLF KUCHER . . . Department of Anaesthesiology,
University of Vienna,
Vienna (Austria)

PETER LAWIN . . . . Department of Anaesthesiology,
University Clinics of Hamburg,
Hamburg (Germany)

IIELENE MAYER . . . . Department of Anesthesiology,
New York University,
New York (U.S.A.)

GABRIEL NAHAS . . . . Department of Anesthesiology,
Columbia University,
New York (U.S.A.)

VLADIMIR NEGOVSKY . . Laboratory of Experimental Physiology
for Resuscitation,
Moscow (U.S.S.R.)

HENNING POULSEN . . . Department of Anaesthesiology,
University of Aarhus,
Aarhus (Denmark)

PETER SAFAR . . . . . Department of Anesthesiology,
University of Pittsburgh,
Pittsburgh (U.S.A.)

MARTIN ZINDLER . . . Department of Anaesthesiology,
Medical Academy of Duesseldorf,
Duesseldorf (Germany)

Introduction. Public health aspects

Safar (Chairman): Ladies and gentlemen, the purpose of this symposium is to have some of the controversial questions in the field of resuscitation discussed informally by an international group. I will first introduce to you the panel of speakers: to my right, Dr. ERNEST KERN, Anesthesiologist of the Hospitals of Paris. To my left, first, Dr. RUDOLF KUCHER of the Department of Anesthesiology, University of Vienna; next, Dr. VLADIMIR NEGOVSKY of the Laboratory of Experimental Physiology for Resuscitation, Moscow, U.S.S.R.; next, Dr. LEROY HARRIS of the Department of Anesthesiology, University of Pittsburgh School of Medicine, U.S.A.; next, Dr. HELENE MAYER of the Department of Anesthesiology, New York University School of Medicine, U.S.A.; next, Dr. PETER LAWIN of the Department of Anesthesiology, University Clinics of Hamburg, Germany; next, Dr. MARTIN ZINDLER of the Department of Anesthesiology, Medical Academy of Duesseldorf, Germany; and lastly, Dr. HENNING POULSEN of the Department of Anesthesiology, University of Aarhus, Denmark.

Each one of the speakers can contribute from his own personal experience with resuscitation which he obtained either in the laboratory or during actual resuscitations of humans or both.

Dr. JAMES JUDE of the Department of Surgery, Johns Hopkins Hospital, Baltimore, Maryland, U.S.A., who is co-author of the pioneering recent publications on external cardiac compression, had planned to participate in this symposium. He wrote me that unexpectedly it turned out to be impossible for him to come to Vienna. He sends his best regards to the panel members and the audience and he asked me to present the data and views of the Johns Hopkins group, whenever applicable.

I would like to invite audience participation during the discussions, as there are some in the audience who have expert knowledge in this field. I would like you to keep questions and comments as brief as possible. The members of the panel decided to speak English. The comments of Dr. NEGOVSKY will be translated. I would like to ask you to speak loudly, slowly and distinctly.

No attempts will be made to discuss any topic in its entirety. There will be no formal papers presented.

Now I want to introduce this symposium with a few comments of my own concerning resuscitation as a Public Health problem (Table 1).

Table 1. *Estimated annual death rates in the U.S.A.*
Conditions in which death sometimes is reversible by resuscitation.

(A) *Accidents*			Total	89,350 (1959) [1]
This includes: [2]			or	91,500 (1961) [2]
	Traffic	38,000		
	Falls	18,400		
	Fires	6,900		
	Drowning	6,550		
	Railroad	2,300		
	Firearms	2,300		
	Poisons	1,800		
	Gas	1,050		
(B) *Arteriosclerotic heart disease*		(Coronary disease)		476,980 (1959) [1]
(C) Surgical deaths with *anesthesia* contribution				
		Avg. 6.6 : 10,000		10,000 [15, 16, 17]
(D) *Maternal* deaths, [18] (1946—1958) 4 Million births				
	Anesthesia	1.2 : 10,000		480
	Hemorrhage	2.2 : 10,000		880
(E) *Neonatal* deaths				69,355 [1]
(F) *Medical* emergencies		Total		?
		Respiratory infection		57,320 [1]
		Total	over	700,000 (approx. 42% of total estimated deaths in U.S.A.)
Total number of deaths in U.S.A. (1959)				1,659,000 [1]

The number of deaths which are possibly reversible by modern respiratory and cardiac resuscitation exceeds that of many infectious diseases. In the U.S.A., the National Health Education Committee [1] reported for the year 1959 approximately 90,000 accidental deaths. Among the 91,500 accidental deaths reported by the Red Cross for 1961 [2], approximately 6,550 were due to drowning, over 3,000 due to other types of accidental asphyxia (e. g. mechanical asphyxiation, poisoning, electric shock), and 38,000 were the results of traffic accidents.

Many of these highway deaths are due to severe head injury, severe crushing injury of the chest or massive blood loss, which often require correction of airway obstruction and artificial ventilation at the scene of the accident and continuance of resuscitative efforts during transportation. On arrival in the hospital, special techniques such as prolonged intermittent positive pressure ventilation, rapid blood replacement and hypothermia may be life-saving. It is not generally recognized that in many of these accidents, the lethal or life-threatening condition can be reversed by modern resuscitation. For instance, few physicians realize that in many cases of head injury with unconsciousness, the vicious cycle which causes cerebral edema and death may be initiated by upper airway soft tissue obstruction, which may be caused merely by mal-positioning of the head [3, 4] and by restlessness with straining, coughing and laryngospasm. Partially obstructed breathing leads to swelling of the brain by virtue of increased jugular vein pressure, lowered arterial oxygen tension and increased arterial carbon dioxide tension [5, 6].

In addition to these 90,000 accidental deaths, there are in the United States almost 500,000 deaths per year due to coronary artery disease. These offer a great challenge for resuscitation specialists, particularly for those responsible for the organization and teaching of lay personnel. With the almost universal acceptance of mouth-to-mouth resuscitation [7] and the recent introduction of external cardiac compression [8], it became possible to start effective cerebral oxygenation in the pulseless patient anywhere, not only in the hospital. The possibility of having the first phase of cardio-pulmonary resuscitation started by a bystander, who most often is a layman, arouses much community interest. This should make us physicians give more thought to this problem.

Most successful reversals of cardiac arrests reported in the literature occurred in the operating rooms. BECK and LEIGHNINGER reported successful revival of 9 patients with fatal heart attacks, which occurred in the hospital outside of the operating rooms [9]. Several of these patients are now, several years after the cardiac arrest, alive and well. These patients had proven ventricular fibrillation and were resuscitated with ventilation, thoracotomy, internal (direct) cardiac compressions and defibrillation. There have been more cases of this type since the introduction of external cardiac compression.

In the past, a lethal heart attack has been a hopeless situation. It would be of interest to learn how many patients who suffered cardiac arrest outside the operating rooms from what seems to be coronary occlusion, and who had proven ventricular fibrillation or asystole, have been saved up to date. By "saved", I mean have been reversed to the pre-arrest status of body and cerebral function. There were 5 such heart attack patients completely revived by the Johns Hopkins group [10], 2 at the Baltimore City Hospital [11], where I had worked in the past, 5 at the Presbyterian-University Hospital of

Pittsburgh (in one year), and 6 I know of in various other institutions. In the experience of the University of Pittsburgh and the Johns Hopkins resuscitation teams only about 10% of the resuscitation attempts in patients with fatal heart attack led to complete recovery to the pre-arrest status. We hope that this salvage of cardiac patients in hospitals can be improved by better in-service training of all physicians and nurses. Telemonitoring of all cardiac patients may provide the resuscitation alarm and the start of resuscitation to occur sooner following the onset of cardiac arrest.

How many successful reversals of lethal heart attacks outside of the operating room do you know of?

Kern: Two cases.

Negovsky: Four cases.

Mayer: There were two such cases at the New York University Hospitals.

Zindler: I know of two such patients with coronary death.

Poulsen: One case.

Holmdahl: Two patients of the specified type have been saved at the University of Uppsala.

Keszler: I have no personal experience or knowledge of successful resuscitation of coronary heart attacks outside the operating room.

Safar: ADELSON and HOFFMANN [12] of Cleveland performed autopsies on 500 unselected patients who suffered what clinically seemed to have been sudden lethal heart attacks. 63% of these hearts examined showed no evidence of recent coronary artery or myocardial lesions. In addition, the animal investigations of LEIGHNINGER and BECK [13] suggest that some of the patients whose hearts stop suddenly may be resuscitable. We believe that these hearts are probably thrown into ventricular fibrillation by temporary ischemia of the myocardium (localized or diffuse), possibly due to coronary spasm. This may be without permanent impairment of myocardial contractility if fibrillation is reversed.

In addition to these accidents and heart attacks, I want to mention an estimated 10,000 surgical deaths each year in the United States in which anesthesia contributed to the death of the patient. This anesthesia mortality figure is an estimate, based on approximately 15,000,000 anesthetics per year and the assumption that an average of 6.6 in 10,000 anesthesias contributes to the death of the patient. The Baltimore Joint Anesthesia Study Committee, for instance [14, 15], which is reviewing all surgical deaths in a community of approximately 2,000,000 people, found that in approximately 4 of 10,000 operations, the anesthetic management contributed to the death of the patient. In a study of DRIPPS and associates [16], this ratio was approximately 20—40 in 10,000. In a study of BEECHER and TODD [17], it was approximately 6.6 in 10,000 and in a study of another large teaching institution, it was approximately 20 in 10,000. The difference in these figures can probably be explained on the basis of a difference in the physical status of the patients who had surgery in these institutions and in a difference of the methods of evaluation of the contribution of anesthesia to the death.

The *prevention* of these anesthesia associated deaths seems to be primarily a problem of training more expert personnel. The *treatment* of serious anesthetic accidents lies in proper resuscitation. In the final analysis, all anesthetic deaths are due to inadequate resuscitation.

Mothers are dying because of pregnancy and childbirth at a rate of approximately 8.8 per 10,000 live births [18]. Hemorrhage (2.2 per 10,000), infection (1.4 per 10,000), anesthesia (1.2 per 10,000) and toxemia (1 per 10,000) were the principal contributors to maternal mortality in the U.S.A. since 1946 [18].

Finally, I want to mention an unknown number of deaths due to medical emergencies, which are occurring frequently in hospitals, e. g. status asthmaticus, convulsive states, pneumonia and toxemia. Many of these conditions would be reversible with improved and more prompt resuscitation. This statement is based on our own experience with medical emergencies in 2 large teaching institutions.

Now I would like to ask the panel members whether similar data on numbers of accidental deaths are available for other countries.

Zindler: In Germany in 1959, 13,500 people died in 327,000 traffic accidents [19]. The total number of accidental deaths in Germany was approximately 70,000. This does not include deaths due to heart attacks.

Other Members of the Panel: We have no such data available.

Safar: It is apparently very difficult to obtain valid figures. I would like to encourage studies on a community-wide basis similar to those conducted by the Baltimore Joint Anesthesia Study Committee under the Chairmanship of my present associate, PHILLIPS. This committee attempted to evaluate at least all surgery connected deaths within a community, by a group of medical specialists. The protocols are kept anonymous, but the case discussions and the decision concerning the cause of death are by open discussion.

Definition and recognition of cardiac arrest

Safar: Now I would like to ask you how you would define "cardiac arrest".

Poulsen: In this symposium we must consider cardiac arrest not only in the operating theater and in the hospital, but also in emergencies outside the hospital. This means, that when talking to lay people we must use very simple terms in describing a patient with cardiac arrest. What I usually say in such a case about a person who has cardiac arrest is that the patient is gray, pulseless and has wide pupils. Most people with cardiac arrest have dilated pupils.

Safar: Would you agree that cardiac arrest is "the clinical picture of cessation of circulation in a patient who was not expected to die at the time?" This does not include the seriously ill patient who is dying with incurable disease.

Poulsen: Yes, we can use this term.

Harris: This should be slightly qualified by saying that people with heart block (Stokes Adams Syndrome), who have cessation of circulation, may present exceptions. In these patients not all these signs may be present, because of the suddenness of the onset of cessation of circulation. Also, we know that the hearts of these heart block patients may unexpectedly stop. However, we hope to detect this immediately and re-start the heart before brain damage can occur.

Negovsky: I agree with the definition which Dr. SAFAR gave. Maybe it would be suitable to expand this definition to consider cardiac arrest as a case in which the heart still *could* function, but ceased to beat, without having all possibilities of cardiac function lost. As long as the heart is still able to beat, we can call it "cardiac arrest". When the heart stops and is not able to beat, it is the end point of the agonal state.

Safar: I would like to ask Dr. NEGOVSKY to define the "agonal state".

Negovsky: The "agonal state" is the state which precedes clinical death. From the physiopathological point of view the agonal state must be considered as a last "flash" of the active bulbar regulative function during the period of complete extinction (cessation) of the activity of the higher nervous centers. The minimum circulation and respiration which are still persisting during the agonal state do not provide all the vital requirements of an organism. In a long-lasting agonal state there is no chance for successful resuscitation. If the time from the beginning of the first pathological factor influencing the organism until the end of the agonal state lasts up to

10—12 minutes, it is easier to resuscitate successfully. It is very important to pay attention to this deterioration in the "agonal state" in order to start therapy early.

Kern: Cardiac arrest in the clinical term is not always identical with absolute cardiac standstill. Sometimes the heart may beat but absolutely inefficiently. There may be the clinical picture of cessation of circulation even if there is no proof of ventricular fibrillation or asystole.

Safar: I would like to ask the panel members what clinical signs they use to determine cessation of circulation.

Kern: This depends on where it happens. If it happens in the surgical theater in a patient with an open thorax, there is no difficulty in diagnosing cardiac arrest because you see the heart either in asystole or in ventricular fibrillation. In the other cases, there are the signs of the picture which Dr. POULSEN has described: The patient who is apneic, pulseless and gray and whose pupils become wider. It is the clinical picture with which every physician is familiar. Having cardiac arrest diagnosed by laymen is a different problem, which we probably will discuss later.

Safar: How would you teach a layman to detect cessation of circulation?

Kern: I do not think I could do it better than by describing what I have just done. There is no use to listen to heart sounds. The heart may even be beating very feebly, but this is of no practical significance. If you told a layman to feel a pulse, he may not be able to find a pulse. I would describe to the layman cardiac arrest as the picture of a person who is not breathing, who is pale or gray and cold, and whose pupils are dilated.

Safar: We feel that pulselessness of the large arteries is the cardinal sign in diagnosing cardiac arrest. In addition, there should be apnea (or apneustic terminal gasps) and certainly unconsciousness. We do not want to wait for dilatation of the pupils. There is evidence that it may take up to 1 minute before the pupils start dilating, although it may take only 6 seconds from the moment of complete cessation of cerebral circulation to the onset of unconsciousness [20]. We would like to start artificial circulation, if possible, before the pupils dilate. We would certainly have to find out whether laymen are capable of differentiating between presence and absence of a carotid pulse. We have no such evidence at this time, but we are beginning to study the diagnostic capability of laymen.

Negovsky: I agree with what has been said. The signs I would stress are absence of carotid artery pulsations, dilatation of the pupils, areflexia and the color of the patient; in addition, the absence of respiration or the presence of agonal gasps. All these are sufficient signs to show that there is no circulation. Do not bother to take an electrocardiogram as you would lose time. It does not matter if it is a cardiac standstill or ventricular fibrillation, since it is necessary to start resuscitation immediately in both cases.

Holmdahl: You should not wait the 50 seconds that it takes for the pupils to dilate before you start resuscitation. It is also important to know that in acute ventricular fibrillation it may take 2 minutes after complete cessation of circulation before apnea occurs.

Safar: Would you agree if we say "apnea or gasping respirations?"

Holmdahl: Yes, or perhaps better "apnea or changed respirations".

Kern: I had one case of a patient who was admitted with cardiac standstill. We ventilated him and performed cardiac massage for 5 hours. During this period, we tried defibrillation, stimulation with an artificial pacemaker and the injection of drugs (nor-epinephrine, calcium and THAM).

His color improved quickly and the initially dilated pupils contracted. When after 5 hours there was no sign of recovery of the heart, we decided to stop resuscitation. Nevertheless, the patient started breathing spontaneously and we started resuscitation again. We continued for another 2 hours without restoring spontaneous circulation. When again we gave up he continued to breathe without any heart beat for 15 minutes.

Safar: This is very interesting.

Of all organ systems, the central nervous system is most vulnerable to anoxia. Although the brain weighs only 2% of the total body weight, it gets normally about 20% of the blood flow and total oxygen consumption. The cerebral cortex is more vulnerable than the medulla and the spinal cord. Other organs are more resistant to anoxia.

Dr. NEGOVSKY, within how long a period of complete cessation of circulation must artificial ventilation and circulation be started, if irreversible brain damage is to be avoided. Do you have information on dogs and man?

Negovsky: I have no additional ideas on the subject. I agree with what was said. Nothing can be said unless one knows how long the individual has been dead. If the death has been sudden, 5 or 6 minutes may elapse and one can still revive a dog. A human may go for approximately 3 to 4 minutes. A young human being can go as long as 6 minutes. If it is a slow dying process, it is better to start treatment before clinical death occurs. It is known that under such conditions the irreversible changes, particularly those in the brain, may develop already after 1 minute or less of clinical death.

Safar: The 3 to 5 minute interval we are taught is a theoretical one. We actually do not know how long complete cessation of circulation can be tolerated by the human brain, even if normal oxygenation would have been present up to the point of arrest.

Mayer: I think the time interval is variable.

Safar: Do you all agree that in some instances of death from asphyxia, the brain may be irreversibly damaged already before the heart stops, if the individual had a healthy heart to start with?

Several Panel Members: Yes.

Zindler: When we get to the scene of the accident, we usually do not know how long the heart had stopped.

Kern: I think we have few clinical data about this subject, except for cases of thoracic surgery, because we can usually not determine clinically and record the exact time when the heart had stopped. This lack of knowledge is the reason for the discrepancy in the textbooks.

Safar: I think it was clearly shown that the hesitation and the waiting period before opening the chest was the greatest deficiency of the open cardiac massage method. This has been greatly improved by the introduction of external cardiac compression.

A Plan of Action

Safar: I would now like to go into discussing various aspects of resuscitation techniques. As a crutch for our memory, I have listed alphabetically the steps of cardiopulmonary resuscitation (Table 2).

Safar: We should rehearse mentally resuscitative action approximately in this sequence:

(A) Airway.

(B) Breathing (namely, emergency artificial ventilation).

(C) Circulation (namely, artificial circulation).

A, B and C are *Phase I* of resuscitation, which is to re-establish cerebral oxygenation within seconds. Mouth-to-mouth resuscitation and external cardiac compression ideally can be applied anywhere. We still have to learn whether or not laymen can detect cardiac arrest and can apply external cardiac compression without producing unnecessary injury.

Phase II of resuscitation consists of:

(D) Drugs (epinephrine, vasopressors and alkalinizing drugs, e. g. sodium bicarbonate or THAM).

(E) Electrocardiography and electric defibrillation, if necessary.
(F) Fluids (to prime the pump).

Phase II of resuscitation is to re-establish spontaneous circulation. We are not certain at this time whether Phase II should be limited

Table 2. *Phases of resuscitation*

Methods			Personnel to be trained			
			Lay public	Para-med. pers.	M. D.	M. D. Resusc. specialist
Phase I. Emergency oxygenation of Central Nervous System	(A) *Airway:* Backward tilt of head Clearing of pharynx Separation of lips and teeth Positive pressure (e. g. M-M)		×	×	×	×
	Forward displacement of mandible			×	×	×
	Pharyngeal tube			×	×	×
	Tracheal tube or cricothyroid membrane puncture				×	×
	(B) *Breathing:* Mouth to mouth Mouth to nose		×	×	×	×
	Mouth to adjunct (tube or mask)			×	×	×
	Bag (Bellows)-mask			×	×	×
	(C) *Circulation:* Recognition of cardiac arrest External cardiac compression		?	?	×	×
	Open chest cardiac compression				?	×
Phase II. Restoration of spon-taneous circulation	(D) *Drugs:* Epinephrine Norepinephrine Sodium Bicarbonate				×	×
	(E) *EKG:* Defibrillation				×	×
	(F) *Fluids:* Saline Plasma expander Blood				×	×

Table 2. (continued)

Methods		Personnel to be trained			
		Lay public	Para-med. pers.	M. D.	M. D. Resusc. specialist
Phase III.	(G) Gauging (should efforts be continued?)				×
Long-Term Resuscitation	(H) *Hypothermia*				×
	(I) *Intensive Care:* Tracheotomy Mechanical artificial ventilation Care of unconscious patient Correction of cause of arrest Inhalation therapy				×

to medical personnel or whether para-medical personnel could be trained to inject epinephrine, or to apply an external electric defibrillating shock.

We found no step in resuscitation which starts with "G", so we may call it "gauging". This means: determination of salvability — namely, whether resuscitation efforts should be continued or abandoned.

Phase III of resuscitation consists of:

(H) Hypothermia (to minimize cerebral edema and the inflammatory response of the brain to the anoxic insult following arrest), and

(I) Intensive Care (consisting of tracheotomy, prolonged artificial ventilation, fluid balance and the general patient care).

Phase III of resuscitation is "long-term resuscitation". This phase, because of the many complicated methods involved, should certainly be limited to the hospital and should be performed by specialized resuscitation teams, preferably in Intensive Care Units.

Phases I and II are non-specific and usually do not require the diagnosis of the cause of death, since the techniques to be applied are practically identical, regardless of the cause of cardiac arrest. There are a few exceptions, for instance, air embolism, pneumothorax, cardiac tamponade, etc. Phase III, however, should include the diagnosis of the cause of death and the treatment should not only be aimed at reversing the dying process "per se", but also to correct the underlying disease process.

A. Airway

Safar: Dr. POULSEN, could you please give us a brief outline of how you would teach lay personnel to recognize and treat airway obstruction?

Poulsen: In emergency resuscitation, diagnosis and treatment of airway obstruction are of great importance. Any anesthetist knows this, but anesthetists are not always present when accidents occur which result in loss of consciousness, airway obstruction and asphyxia.

Diagnosis and simple treatment of airway obstruction must therefore be taught to any potential rescuer, i. e. to the public at large.

Instructions to lay people must be short, accurate, extremely simple and easy to remember.

In the unconscious victim, the diagnosis of airway obstruction must be based on the simple fact that obstruction prevents air from going in and out of the chest. If the chest does not move up and down, obstruction must be suspected — and the airway must be opened by backward tilt of the head and, possibly, by clearing the pharynx.

Safar: Doesn't the chest move up and down also when there is paradoxic movement with airway obstruction in the spontaneously breathing patient?

Poulsen: This is quite right but it does not give the up and down movement of the chest I am referring to.

Safar: You mean in obstruction, the chest is going "down and up" instead of "up and down".

Poulsen: Yes, down and slightly up, combined with retraction of the jugular fossa during the inspiratory downward movement of the chest.

Physicians, nurses and rescue personnel can be taught to distinguish between airway obstruction in the spontaneously breathing patient and the apneic patient by inspection of the suprasternal area, etc., but laymen may be confused if more elaborate diagnostic measures are required.

If the chest is moving up and down in a normal manner, the airway obstruction cannot be extensive. We should teach the lay personnel, as a primary measure, to tilt the head backward and, if necessary, to remove mucus or other foreign matter from the pharynx. As far as obstruction is concerned, they will see whether these maneuvers have changed the movements of the chest.

Safar: In the training of lay personnel, would you add to the simple backward tilt of the head also forward displacement of the mandible, the second but more difficult step? I am referring to the lay public at large, not to para-medical personnel such as nurses or ambulance personnel.

Poulsen: I would not add forward displacement of the mandible because it may be too complicated to teach and to learn. The same applies to the use of pharyngeal tubes.

Safar: Would you teach forward displacement of the mandible, to paramedical personnel?

Poulsen: Yes, I have done this already for several years.

Safar: Would you also teach the insertion of pharyngeal tubes to paramedical personnel?

Poulsen: Yes, certainly. The use of pharyngeal tubes and forward displacement of the mandible should be taught to para-medical personnel, nurses and doctors.

Safar: Would you agree that — if backward tilt of the head alone did not correct airway obstruction — one should try to overcome this obstruction by adding positive pressure inflation attempts, even in the presence of spontaneous breathing movements? Positive pressure can often overcome obstruction.

Poulsen: Yes, I certainly agree.

Safar: In summary then, we agree that we should teach all people backward tilt of the head in the unconscious patient [3, 4]. If this does not lead to air exchange, positive pressure inflation should be used in addition. Paramedical personnel should also learn forward displacement of the mandible and insertion of a pharyngeal tube as additional maneuvers if necessary.

This leads us now to techniques which are more elaborate, namely, the use of *tracheal intubation* and *tracheotomy*.

How do you feel about tracheotomy vs. oro-tracheal intubation vs. crico-thyroid membrane puncture in the hands of physicians?

Poulsen: In my opinion, tracheal intubation has a place in resuscitation in the field, but two conditions must be fulfilled: first, skilled personnel must be present; and secondly, equipment. By "skilled personnel", I mean a person of any category (physician, nurse or professional rescuer) who had a thorough training in the technical procedure of tracheal intubation.

Safar: Would you agree that tracheal intubation should only be considered if previous attempts at inflating the lungs without a tracheal tube had failed?

Poulsen: Yes. Quite a few doctors are not specialists in resuscitation or tracheal intubation. We may disagree but I feel that all doctors, including general practitioners should know how to perform tracheal intubation. Anyway, the skilled person and the equipment must be available if tracheal intubation should be tried at all.

Has tracheotomy any place in emergency resuscitation? I should say hardly any. This procedure takes quite a long time and is distracting in an emergency. A tracheal tube should always be inserted, if possible, before tracheotomy is performed. This means that we already have a safe airway established before starting the tracheotomy procedure.

Complete airway obstruction by an unremovable foreign body may occur although it is relatively rare, and in such cases, puncture of the crico-thyroid membrane must be the method of choice.

Safar: Who among the panel members or the audience has had experience with crico-thyroid membrane puncture?

Has anybody ever punctured the crico-thyroid membrane, using a knife, trocar or large bore needle?

Kern: I remember a patient who had a fracture of the mandible and bled for some hours into the trachea. While I was trying to clean the airway, the surgeon punctured the crico-thyroid membrane and we got the patient through.

Safar: It is interesting that his method, which is mentioned in most textbooks has never been applied by this group of specialists.

Member of the Audience: This is because we are all anesthetists who know how to pass tracheal tubes. I have seen a case with obstruction of the tracheal tube treated successfully by insufflating oxygen via a needle, inserted through the crico-thyroid membrane or the trachea.

Safar: Did the oxygen get into the trachea or into the mediastinum?

Member of the Audience: The trachea was insufflated and the patient is still alive.

Mayer: We had a patient who required crico-thyroid membrane puncture with a 15 gauge needle until tracheostomy could be done. The patient was successfully resuscitated. Unfortunately, the esophagus was perforated by the procedure.

Member of the Audience: I have tried a cannula of 3 mm. diameter, inserted through the crico-thyroid membrane and adapted it to a Ruben resuscitator. It worked beautifully for producing artificial ventilation.

Safar: 3 mm. is a large bore which is probably adequate. A 13 gauge needle, commonly recommended, may permit emergency re-oxygenation in adults only if oxygen is insufflated in high flow rates. In addition, the patient must either have spontaneous breathing movements or artificial *intermittent* insufflation of oxygen must be used for artificial ventilation. The needle without oxygen is not adequate for long periods of spontaneous breathing or for artificial ventilation with air or exhaled air insufflation.

Member of the Audience: I agree.

Holmdahl: Once the lungs have been inflated a few times with pure oxygen, it becomes possible to sustain life for many minutes by insufflation via a small tracheal needle behind an upper airway obstruction, even with a low flow rate of oxygen, thus maintaining "apneic diffusion oxygenation" [21].

Safar: The ensuing hypercarbia then certainly must be corrected as soon as possible by ventilation via an adequate airway.

Proper "plumbing", namely, inserting tubes and connecting these tracheal tubes to resuscitation equipment, is a common difficulty with tracheotomies in emergency resuscitation. Although crico-thyroid membrane puncture may be an emergency procedure, as it can be more rapidly performed than a tracheotomy, it may be difficult to ventilate the apneic patient through a relatively small bore needle or trocar. Therefore, because of lack of "plumbing", we should always try some other method first, namely, inflating the lungs with positive pressure through the mouth or nose. The relative role of each of these techniques in a given location depends on the training of the personnel available.

B. Breathing

Emergency artificial ventilation

Safar: I would like to skip over the topic of emergency artificial ventilation rapidly, unless there are disagreements, since much has been said and written during recent years about exhaled air ventilation and other positive pressure methods. It has been shown that in the absence of equipment, intermittent positive pressure ventilation with exhaled air, preferably without the use of adjuncts, is the method of choice [22, 23, 24]. By this, I mean direct mouth-to-mouth and mouth-to-nose ventilation.

Methods which rely upon compression and expansion of the thorax are not as reliable because of lack of control over the airway (lack of support of the head and jaw), the inability to determine adequacy of ventilation and the inability to adapt the inflation pressures to the pulmonary resistance (i. e. airway resistance plus lung-thorax compliance), which changes dynamically during emergency artificial ventilation [23, 25].

Now, I would like to get away from the field conditions, which require artificial ventilation without equipment, and ask Mr. DENNY from Australia, who has had great experience as a lay instructor of rescue squads, whether hand-operated equipment such as bag-mask units or bellows units offer any advantage over the use of mechanical resuscitators in ambulances.

Denny (Instructor, Royal Life-Saving Society, Melbourne, Australia): This is a touchy subject as far as lay personnel is concerned. Before we go any further, you have to re-evaluate the knowledge of the layman. You put him too far down on the scale of intelligence. In some aspects of resuscitation, a layman could actually give you lessons concerning the first treatment of the patient, because we are the first on the scene of the accident. We, in Australia, have special instructional units which teach the general public, beginning at the age of 8 years. The people are taught mouth-to-mouth and mouth-to-nose ventilation, closed-chest heart massage and also mouth-to-nose in water rescues. The grade of instruction is adapted to the average of the group. The more advanced the group, the more knowledge they are given. What we are talking about today, we have published in our handbook of the Royal Life-Saving Society of Australia (Royal Life-Saving Society: V.C.A. Building, Melbourne, Australia).

We have been teaching these methods for about 2 years. We are teaching prevention as well as cure.

In regards to machines in ambulances, too much attention is given to the machine and not to the patient. The first rescuer may get the patient under control, breathing adequately, then the machine is used incorrectly and the patient is dead on arrival. We feel that the bag type of resuscitator would focus the operator's attention back to the care of the patient, and not on the machine, as it so often happens. We discourage the use of mechanical equipment in the hands of those who do not quite know what to do with it.

Safar: There is plenty of evidence that during emergency resuscitation ventilation has to be adapted to the changing resistances and air leaks, which requires a breath-to-breath control of inflation pressure, -volume, -flow and rate. This control is not possible with the use of automatic cycling resuscitators, but it is possible with the use of hand-operated equipment and with the use of your own lungs.

Poulsen: We have considered this problem for several years and all our ambulances are equipped with hand-operated resuscitators, viz. Ruben bags. We have no mechanical ventilators of any kind in the hands of ambulance personnel in Denmark.

Zindler: I wonder whether the layman may not do better with the use of his own lungs, using equipment with a mouth piece for the patient and a large corrugated tubing with special valves (Seeler valve), like the oro-resuscitator or other adjuncts for exhaled air ventilation. This may be better in this respect than the Ruben bag or the bellows. For a layman, it is much easier to get a proper fit with this equipment and there is a larger reserve volume available.

Safar: I would like to ask Dr. NEGOVSKY how he feels about the use of *oxygen* for use in emergency artificial ventilation, assuming that oxygen is available. Dr. NEGOVSKY has published in the past, statements implying that high oxygen tensions should be avoided in resuscitation.

Negovsky: This question is not as simple as it many imply. One certainly should give oxygen first. However, after a severe and prolonged hypoxia, for instance, after 10—15 minutes of dying caused by hemorrhage, followed by 5—6 minutes of clinical death, oxygen may become occasionally harmful. When not as profound and long-lasting a hypoxia preceded death, for instance, 1 to 2 minutes after a sudden cardiac arrest, oxygen is indicated. I would like to state once more the basis of this question. During prolonged dying with prolonged hypotension, and deep hypoxia, it is better and more "gentle" if you use a mixture of air and oxygen. So, if there has been profound hypoxia, it is better to give a mixture of oxygen and air, not more than 40% oxygen.

Safar: Does this hold true for both emergency resuscitation attempts as well as prolonged artificial ventilation?

Negovsky: This answer concerns emergency resuscitation.

Safar: If you use pure oxygen in a deeply cyanotic person, in order to re-oxygenate him rapidly, what harmful effects would you see from the use of oxygen in such a case, as compared to re-oxygenation with air?

Negovsky: Physiologic studies have shown that during resuscitation following prolonged and profound hypoxia, the oxygen acts poisonous on nerve cells. Pathologic findings after prolonged periods of profound hypoxia have shown that there is a toxic effect on brain cells following the use of pure oxygen. There is a state of well pronounced hypoxia during the period of dying, during clinical death and during the post-resuscitation period. It would appear quite natural, therefore, to use at that time oxygen therapy. A number of authors [26—32] though point out the high sensitivity to oxygen of an organism suffering from deep hypoxia and the paradoxic effect, namely, *hyperoxia,* produced by pure oxygen under these conditions [33].

The investigations made in our laboratory have shown that after 5 minutes of clinical death from hemorrhage, only 4 of 40 dogs, which had been treated with pure oxygen, revived. In contrast, there were as many as 50% and more survivors in the control group. However, recent investigations on the topic have shown the great significance of the cause of death and of the state of hemodynamics during resuscitation. Thus, in our experiments with prolonged external massage for the sudden cardiac arrest caused by electrocution, the best results have been obtained with the use of pure oxygen [34].

Safar: How do you differentiate the brain cell changes caused by the high oxygen tension from those caused by the hypoxia itself?

Negovsky: The toxic effect of the pure oxygen in a state of deep hypoxia is manifested not as much by the changes in the nerve cells, as by its effect on the organism as a whole. The use of 100% O_2 provoked increased vascular permeability. At autopsy, a great many extravasations were found, not only in brain, but in all viscera.

Kucher: Dr. NEGOVSKY, how can we differentiate clinically between hypoxia and anoxia?

Negovsky: It is better to skip all differentiation here. There is almost never a complete anoxia. There is usually only hypoxia.

Safar: These observations of Dr. NEGOVSKY are very interesting because there is evidence that re-oxygenation can be accomplished more rapidly with the use of high oxygen tensions, particularly in patients with abnormal lungs, for instance with diffusion abnormalities, such as pulmonary edema [35]. This particular problem of the abnormal lungs, Dr. NEGOVSKY has not touched upon. We feel, that in most dying patients, the lungs are not normal and re-oxygenation is faster when we use pure oxygen rather than air.

Kern: I understand, Professor NEGOVSKY, that your views are based chiefly on experimental grounds. But in practice, if a patient needs emergency respiratory resuscitation, there often may be some degree of airway obstruction. If you then give 100% oxygen, you get a much better chance for re-oxygenation. Even if you feel from experiments that air-oxygen mixtures may give a better result in emergency resuscitation, in a practical sense the use of pure oxygen gives a better chance for survival.

Negovsky: I agree that in sudden hypoxia you can begin the treatment by giving pure oxygen. But, one should always have in mind that the long-lasting oxygenation with pure oxygen may be occasionally harmful. So, in some cases it probably would be better to switch to air-oxygen mixtures.

Safar: In Professor Woolmer's laboratory in London, some work was done on anesthesia for animals in oligemic shock [36]. It was found that the crucial factor in the survival of these animals was the oxygen tension rather than the anesthetic agent used. The survival rate was higher in the dogs which received air-oxygen mixtures than in the dogs which received air only.

I would like to ask Dr. ZINDLER to comment on what his panel concluded to be evidence of "oxygen toxicity" in resuscitation.

Zindler: There are two possibilities of damage due to high oxygen tensions: firstly, to the brain and secondly, to the lungs. Our symposium discussed only the applications of artificial ventilation in connection with the use of the heart-lung machine. I assume that in situations of emergency resuscitation, oxygen has no chance to get to the brain and other tissues in high enough tensions to create any damage there.

As to the damage to the lungs, the problem is how long can you give pure oxygen to a patient who is mechanically ventilated. It has been our opinion that you should give pure oxygen only for several hours or half a day, but there were two members of our panel who have given mechanical artificial ventilation with pure oxygen for weeks without having observed any apparent damage. I believe, however, that for prolonged artificial ventilation we should give it only if we think that it is really necessary. It depends how much you can get into the tissues with the use of 60% oxygen inhaled, and whether you can get much more in with 100% than with 60%. Usually, there may not be much difference. Certainly, I believe that with the use of up to 60% inhaled oxygen there is no evidence that it can cause harm.

Kern: Does Dr. NEGOVSKY know whether the Russian space travellers who have been in space for over 4 days were exposed to oxygen or oxygen-air mixtures?

Negovsky: I am sorry I have not been there. I am convinced, however, that they were not breathing pure oxygen.

Safar: I had an opportunity to discuss this with Dr. SEVERING-HAUS. He suggested that the overall tension in the space capsule could be kept lower than atmospheric with the use of pure oxygen inhalation. A high concentration of oxygen at low total pressure may give the same inhaled tension as breathing air under normal pressure.

Nahas: In all this, one certainly should talk about oxygen tension at the tissue level and not oxygen tension in the inspired air. What may possibly be damaging is high oxygen tension in the tissues. But in order to have high oxygen tensions in the tissues, one may not need 100% oxygen in the inspired air if the circulation is adequate. But, if the circulation is inadequate, for instance in shock with poor circulation, one will have usually low oxygen tension in the tissues in spite of breathing 100% oxygen.

Safar: Certainly most of us have seen patients ventilated with pure oxygen for several days with complete recovery without any evidence of pulmonary or central nervous system damage. We probably have to accept the fact that there is no answer to this question of oxygen toxicity at this time. There just is not enough available evidence that, in man, pulmonary damage from high inhaled oxygen partial pressures (up to 1 atmosphere) may occur in the presence of adequate humidification. More work has to be done on this subject.

Member of the Audience: We were talking about airway and positive pressure ventilation, but you did not mention anything about *suction*, which is so vital to clear the airway.

Safar: The point is very well taken. Unfortunately, there was not enough time to go into the problems of foreign matter in the upper air passages and inhalation of gastric contents and other material.

Member of the Audience: I would do suctioning before oxygenation.

Zindler: Would you really do suctioning first in the cyanotic patient before you oxygenate him? I do not think anybody here would, unless one sees that the mouth is full of blood or vomitus.

Safar: I think it is agreed that you should attempt to force oxygen into the lungs first when the patient is cyanotic, instead of delaying re-oxygenation by first suctioning [37].

What sort of suction equipment would you recommend for use in ambulances?

Kern: Very simple equipment, which could be handled successfully by laymen. I think, I would discard electrical or mechanical driven suction apparatus in favor of those which are available and can be kept working manually.

Mayer: In the absence of equipment. I would wipe the mouth and pharynx with the fingers and place the patient into the head down position or the lateral position. An Ambu foot pump could be used in ambulances.

Zindler: An Ambu foot-operated suction I would recommend for ambulances.

Poulsen: The question of suctioning equipment for use in ambulances has been discussed in Denmark since 1957, and the result of this discussion is that all ambulances in Denmark are today provided with the following equipment:

1. *A built-in suction unit* in which, in gasoline-driven ambulances, the suction power is derived from the manifold of the engine. This is able to develop a vacuum of 300—400 mm. Hg in a 5 liter reser-

voir placed beside the engine and connected to a suitable suction bottle and catheter.

In diesel-engined ambulances, the suction power is usually provided by an injector arrangement connected to the exhaust tube.

2. *A portable suction device* consisting of Ruben's Ambu suction unit. The latter device is necessary to ensure prompt treatment of patients at the scene of accident, but this does not make the built-in unit superfluous, as the foot-operated Ambu pump is extremely difficult to use during high-speed driving.

Safar: Semi-solid or solid foreign matter can only be cleared satisfactorily from the pharynx by manual wiping. Concerning equipment for clearing liquid foreign matter from the air passages, I agree entirely with Dr. POULSEN on the basis of experience with suction apparatus in ambulances and on the basis of measurements we have performed on flows and vacuums of various suction devices. The oxygen-powered venturi-type suction proved inadequate. ROSEN [38] recommends a maximal vacuum of at least 600 mm. Hg and a flow rate of at least 30 liters per minute.

Harris: I agree with what was recommended.

C. Circulation

External and internal cardiac compression

Safar: Now we are coming to the question of artificial circulation. I would like to ask Dr. LAWIN to present his experience with arterial pressures he observed during external cardiac compression in patients with proven cessation of circulation.

Lawin: In our clinical experience, the effect of external cardiac compression is about the same as that of internal cardiac compression (slide shown). With sternal compressions, we measured artificial arterial pressures in man of up to 160 mm. Hg systolic. The acute angle formed by the return of the pressure curve from the systolic to the diastolic slope is indicative of the aortic valve closure, while the continued increase of the diastolic pressure indicates a continued supply of blood to the arterial and venous system. The assistance to venous return is an advantage of external compression over the direct internal cardiac massage. The return of the wave cushion against the closed aortic valve, as seen particularly in the recording of the pulse curve, is an indication of the air funnel ("Windkessel") function, showing satisfactory output of the left ventricle.

We have measured arterial pressures with the Statham-transducer in 6 patients during cardiac arrest, treated with external cardiac compressions. These were patients after open-heart surgery who developed ventricular fibrillation after closure of the chest. In the same cases, we tried re-thoracotomy and internal defibrillation without success. These badly damaged hearts are very difficult to resuscitate.

Safar: Dr. LAWIN's pressure tracings during external cardiac compression confirm those obtained by the Johns Hopkins group and by our department at the Baltimore City Hospitals in 1959/61 [39]. In eight dying patients, we recorded systolic pressures of between 80 and 160 mm. Hg during external cardiac compression when there was no spontaneous pulse and the electrocardiogram showed ventricular fibrillation or asystole. The diastolic pressures were always extremely low. For obvious reasons, a controlled comparison of the external over the internal method in man is lacking. We have observed 5 patients with no artificial pulse produced by the external method, in whom the chest was subsequently opened and 4 of the 5 patients had an artificial pulse with the performance of the internal method [40].

Does anyone have information on blood flow measurements during external cardiac compression in man?

Members of the Audience and Panel: No.

Safar: There is clinical evidence of blood flow during external cardiac compressions, since reflexes recover, the pupils become smaller, the wound starts bleeding and the patient may start gasping.

Mayer: Consciousness and ability to remember the episode can be restored during external massage. Also, ventricular fibrillation may revert to normal sinus rhythm spontaneously after external massage. We have cases at the Bellevue Hospital of New York to prove these points.

Safar: Now I would like to ask whether you have any comparative data on the mechanical efficacy of external vs. internal cardiac compressions on dogs.

Members of the Audience and Panel: No.

Safar: I would like to mention the work of my former associate, REDDING [41]. He has compared the external and the internal cardiac compression methods in two comparable groups of ten dogs each. During ventricular fibrillation, the artificial arterial pressures and carotid flow rates with either method varied tremendously from dog to dog, between approximately 4 and 40% of the spontaneous control flows. The average flows and pressures with external cardiac compression were about the same as those with thoracotomy and internal cardiac compression. After defibrillation and restoration of effective spontaneous circulation, however, the average arterial pressures and flows were higher in the group treated with the closed technique, possibly because these animals suffered less trauma.

Harris: The artificial flows measured during external cardiac compression (performed with a mechanical chest compressor) measured in our experiments on 50 dogs, ranged between 10 and 30% of the spontaneous flows in the intact anesthetized animals.

Zindler: We have no data on that. It certainly would be difficult to get them in humans. My present opinion is that even in the operating room, if the chest is closed, you should start first with the external massage, but prepare immediately for opening the chest. In about two minutes, you have to decide whether or not you should continue with external compressions. If the patient improves dramatically, there is no use to open the chest. If the patient does not improve in 2 minutes, the chest should be opened in the operating room, as there may be cardiac tamponade, or other conditions which require opening of the chest. In operating room conditions, the open massage should then be used, although it may be more traumatic to the heart.

A great deal depends on the mechanical situation. A disadvantage of the external compression is the possibility of trauma to liver, lungs, heart and ribs. Another disadvantage is that external compression raises considerably the pressure in the great veins (up to 60 cm. of water), which may impair tissue perfusion.

In dogs, the closed massage is much more effective than in a big man with a big chest. I do not think that the methods are in competition, but rather that they supplement each other.

Safar: There is evidence that in dogs thoracotomy and direct manual systole (internal cardiac compression) produces a higher aortic pressure and lower vena cava pressure than external cardiac compressions with the chest intact, suggesting less tissue perfusion with the external method [42].

Negovsky: We have studied internal and external cardiac compression, both in dogs and in the clinic.

With the external compressions, it was possible to maintain the same arterial pressures as with internal compressions.

The hypoxia and the acidosis were much greater under closed chest massage. Nevertheless, when we used the closed method, we could usually restore cardiac activity even if it had been more difficult in some cases than with the open method. In order to restore cardiac contractions in a state of ventricular fibrillation, we had to repeat the defibrillatory electro-shocks 2 to 3 times. As regards the post-resuscitative period, its course has been better with the use of the closed-chest technique [34].

The better resuscitation method is the one which is more rapidly applicable and, therefore, the external method is often more successful. I am in favor of external cardiac compression because you can do it faster and the results, therefore, will be better.

Kucher: The choice between the application of the external and the internal cardiac compression method should be made according to the cause of the cardiac arrest. In my opinion, a reflex cardiac arrest (namely, a vago-vagal cardiac arrest) can probably be reversed without difficulty in most instances with the use of the external method. If there is, however, an anoxic cardiac arrest, the open method will be more successful.

Negovsky: I do not entirely agree with this. We should always start first with the external method with the exception of patients with fractured ribs.

Kern: Dr. KUCHER, you mentioned "vago-vagal" reflex cardiac arrest. Do you really think that such a condition exists in patients?

Kucher: There is no doubt that cardiac arrest can be caused by vago-vagal reflexes [43, 44]. This may be caused by inadequate atropinization, operations on the neck under light anesthesia, particularly in neck infections [45], and manipulations of the hilus of the lung under light anesthesia or with inadequate blockage of reflexes. The hyperactivity of the carotid sinus reflex with subsequent vagal effect on the heart is neither proven nor disproven.

Safar: Do the other panel members feel that vago-vagal cardiac arrest can occur? Does it occur in the oxygenated person or only in the hypoxic person?

Poulsen: I do not know.

Zindler: I do not know either, but in some cases where this is postulated, it may merely be an excuse for some other accident. I do not think this is of great importance. If there is an arrest, you do the same thing about it, whether it is vago-vagal or not. There may be some experimental evidence in dogs that a vago-vagal cardiac arrest can occur, but whether it really can happen in a human is difficult to prove.

Lawin: The question of vago-vagal cardiac arrest is good for the textbooks but not for the practice. I think it is usually an excuse for some other cause.

Mayer: Vago-vagal arrest or glossopharyngeal vagal arrest may occur if there is a hypersensitive carotid sinus [46]. Dr. MAZZIA also has a patient in the Medical Examiner's file who seems to have had vago-vagal cardiac arrest while he apparently was well-oxygenated.

Harris: I do not believe that vago-vagal cardiac arrest can occur in a well-oxygenated man.

Safar: There is evidence certainly that the heart of the hypoxic person can be stopped by stimuli, such as upper airway manipulation during intubation [47]. I know of no evidence whether or not this can happen in the well-oxygenated person. Upper airway stimulation in the well-oxygenated, lightly anesthetized or awake person causes hypertension and tachycardia [48].

Now I would like to ask Dr. HARRIS to tell us something about *how we should combine intermittent positive pressure ventilation with external cardiac compressions.*

Harris: I would like to report the results of our work in dogs [49]. We have attempted to answer certain questions of circulation and ventilation in standardized experiments. In dogs in ventricular fibrillation (produced by external electric shock) external cardiac compressions were kept constant by means of a Beck-Rand heart massage machine and ventilation was maintained at a constant tidal volume of 15 ml./Kg. using room air. The tidal volumes were measured by a Wright Ventilation Meter. The lungs were inflated by means of either a Ruben bag or a piston respirator, the inflation either being interposed between every 2 external cardiac compressions or simultaneous with every second external cardiac compression. Under these conditions, we have studied the effects on aortic pressure, carotid blood flow, tracheal pressure and arterial blood gases.

Simultaneous lung inflations (as compared to interposed lung inflations) caused greater carotid flows in 7 of 15 comparisons, but only in 5 of 15 was this increase of flow over 25% of the control flow. In 5 of 15 comparisons, the flow was the same and in 3 of 15 lower with the simultaneous method as compared to the interposed method. Therefore, there seems to be a slight superiority of the simultaneous type of lung inflation, as far as arterial flows and pressures is concerned. Which type of lung inflation produces better ventilation?

The interposed type of lung inflation gives better ventilation in every instance (Table 3). This became increasingly apparent with longer periods of heart-lung resuscitation. Interposed lung inflations, produced an average oxygen saturation of 92% and a pH of 7.29 at the end of a period of 18 minutes of resuscitation, while the simultaneous type of inflations gave average oxygen saturations of 65% and a pH of 7.16.

In a third series of experiments we attempted to simulate clinical resuscitation by a single operator. We were interested in determining the longest permissible period of uninterrupted external cardiac compressions without lung inflations which would still provide adequate ventilation. During external cardiac compression periods of 15 and 30 seconds, the tracheal tube was clamped to simulate airway obstruction, as it occurs in unconscious man who is not intubated and whose head is not held in the tilted back position [50].

Table 3.

Oxygen saturation and pH during external cardiac compression. Simultaneous versus interposed lung inflations

(5 Dogs, 15 Comparisons).

	Interposed 3 minutes	Simultaneous 3 minutes	Interposed 18 minutes	Simultaneous 18 minutes
Arterial O$_2$ saturation	Avg. 95% (90—99%)	86% (77—95%)	92% (85—100%)	65% (55—87%)
Arterial pH	Avg. 7.47 (7.31—7.63)	7.38 (7.19—7.52)	7.29 (7.13—7.53)	7.16 (7.05—7.29)

Safar: Airway obstruction almost always occurs when a single operator lets the head assume the passive position in order to have his hands free for compression of the sternum. Even when the head was held tilted backward and even when the tracheal tube was in place, we found that not more than dead space ventilation can be produced by sternal pressures alone [50].

Harris: Oxygen saturations were monitored during ventilation/ external cardiac compression ratios of 3/15 and 6/30, at 1 second intervals (Table 4).

Table 4.

Arterial oxygen saturation during external cardiac comperession. Comparison of 3 inflations/ 15 ECC and 6 inflations/30 ECC

(5 Dogs, 15 Comparsions)

	Control	V. F. 1 min. ECC	3/15 6 min.	6/30 6 min.	3/15 18 min.	6/30 18 min.
O$_2$ sat.	Avg. 93% (86—97%)	65% (50—79%)	93% (85—99%)	90% (81—99%)	90% (85—95%)	74% (70—80%)

With the 3/15 ratio at the end of 20 minutes of resuscitation, the average oxygen saturation had dropped from the normal control value of 93% to an average of 90% (lowest 85%). With the 6/30 ratio the oxygen saturation dropped to an average of 74% (lowest 70%) in a comparable period of time. We, therefore, concluded that, when using room air for ventilation, 30 chest compressions without ventilation may be too long, also in humans. The tidal volumes used in these experiments were 3 times the spontaneous tidal volumes of the dog. We chose these volumes because in clinical resuscitation of adults, we use 1,000 to 1,500 ml. tidal volumes from a Ruben bag. The use of three rapid lung inflations alternated with 15 sternal compressions produced adequate ventilation with relatively short periods of interruption of circulation. We recommend this 3/15 ratio for the reasons mentioned above and also because it can be performed by a single operator and is easy to teach.

Safar: Similar experiments were performed by WILDER in Baltimore [51]. He found that the blood flow rates were significantly better when ventilation was simultaneous with sternal compressions. I believe that most of the Americans who worked with these problems, namely, GORDON, JUDE, ELAM and WILDER and our own group agree that one can not go wrong in recommending an alternating performance of *2—3 rapid deep lung inflations with 15 uninterrupted sternal compressions at 1 second intervals.* This technique can be used by 1 or 2 operators. It also gives better circulation than if we would interrupt after every 4 to 5 sternal compressions to ventilate the lungs, as was recommended earlier [50].

In our clinical experience, interposing a breath without a pause after every 4 to 5 sternal compressions is difficult, unless there is a tracheal tube in place. With bag-mask or mouth-to-mouth ventilation, it is almost impossible to inflate the lungs adequately in less than 1 second. Very high inflation pressures would be required, which in the non-intubated subject would lead to gastric insufflation or may be impossible because of air leaks at the subject's face. Interposing ventilation, even in an unco-ordinated fashion, is possible (and we recommend it) once the trachea is intubated. Then ventilation can be carried out without leakage, with high inflation pressures and with the use of oxygen.

I believe that this concept of combining ventilation with circulation may change with time as more work on this subject will be reported.

Dr. HARRIS, you have recently observed the effect of manual pressure over the abdomen to improve artificial circulation. Can you tell us about it?

Harris: This was studied on 6 dogs, 6 determinations each. We compared aortic pressures and carotid flow rates with alternating ventilation 2/1, with the use of the Beck-Rand machine. We alternated periods with and without continuous manual compression of the abdomen. In one instance, there was no change in blood flow when the abdomen was compressed. Once there was only a 10%

increase in blood flow with abdominal compression. In all other cases, however, the blood flow increased over 20⁰/o with abdominal compression.

Safar: Is this caused by splinting the diaphragm and thus the lungs, or is it due to compression of the abdominal aorta?

Harris: It is not due to compression of the abdominal aorta because femoral artery mean pressures increased during abdominal compression simultaneously with the increase of carotid pressures. Two factors seem to cause the increased arterial pressures and flows with abdominal compression: (1.) Splinting of the diaphragm, confining the entire force of sternal compression to the thoracic cavity; and (2.) The prevention of back flow of blood into the inferior vena cava system, which is caused by external cardiac compressions in the absence of increased intra-abdominal pressure.

Safar: GORDON and others felt that we should not teach this maneuver in spite of the improved blood flow, since he has observed ruptures of the liver in dogs with the use of abdominal compression [51].

Harris: Rupture of the liver was observed twice in our series of dogs who had abdominal compression. It has also been observed, however, several times in the other 30 dogs in whom we did not use abdominal compression. I have no evidence whether or not continuous abdominal compression leads more often to rupture of the liver. Continuous abdominal compression may be a worth while clinical maneuver not only to improve blood flow but also to prevent gastric insufflation during ventilation without tracheal tube.

Zindler: One question on the technique of cardiac massage. Are you taking the patient off the bed or do you massage in bed with a board under him?

Safar: There is too much delay trying to move a patient to the floor. On the floor, it is difficult to start an infusion and to ventilate the patient. We first try to obtain an artificial pulse by massaging the patient where he lies and slide a board under him as soon as possible. There is a board on our resuscitation cart.

Holmdahl: We look for constriction of the pupils and improvement of the color. This tells us we are getting peripheral circulation. The danger of causing injury should make the operator compress no more than necessary to produce a palpable peripheral pulse.

In cases of Adams-Stokes syndrome, often only slight mechanical stimulation causes the ventricles to contract spontaneously. If one follows the rule to depress the sternum one to two inches, one may cause unnecessary damage, as it occurred in an old emphysematic patient with complete heart block. He was transported via an ambulance 200 km. under vigorous external heart compressions. When he arrived in the hospital, nearly all ribs were crushed and it was found that the slightest stimulus to the precordium produced a good heart beat.

Zindler: In cardiac arrest where the heart is still able to beat, the mechanical stimulus of external compression may elicit a strong spontaneous contraction. We have seen this in a child in whom an arterial pressure recording suggested that each sternal compression was followed by a spontaneous contraction.

Safar: In these patients one usually fractures the ribs at the costochondral junction. It is difficult in middle-aged and old patients to produce a palpable peripheral pulse without causing costochondral separations. Although, in our experience, this is common, I know of only one patient in whom the flail chest required treatment. Usually, the pleura is not pierced by these fractures.

Safar: Are there any other comments on injuries caused by external cardiac compression?

Kern: I know of several cases of rib fractures, one of my personal experience.

Zindler: We have also seen rib fractures in two cases.

Safar: I know of 2 cases of internal injuries found at autopsy, one a rupture of the liver and one a hematoma of the mediastinum, which may not have been compatible with survival, although in these instances the patients were not resuscitable when found. In our patients who came to autopsy, we have not seen internal injuries other than rib fractures.

There has been bone marrow embolism observed in the lungs. It is questionable whether this is due to external cardiac compression, since such emboli are also seen in cases of trauma not connected with external cardiac compression. Are there any other comments?

Lawin: We have also seen fractures of the ribs. We feel that the injury is caused by the use of 2 hands. Together with RITTMEYER we have modified this method. Usually the external cardiac massage with one hand in the direction of the output of the left ventricle is sufficient. The other hand is lying over the femoral artery to monitor the effect of the compressions. The effect of external cardiac massage does not depend on excessive force, but on the direction of the force. The soft, but strong compression of the sternum during systole is followed by a quick release of the manual pressure. The sternum is reaching its normal position and so causes a negative intrathoracic pressure, which increases venous backflow to the heart. We believe that a frequency of 60 per minute with a palpable femoral pulse is sufficient for restoring good diastolic filling of the ventricles. Inadequate application of the external cardiac massage (too much force, parasternal compression) may produce rib fractures, rupture of the spleen and liver, etc. These injuries can be avoided.

Kucher: We have seen in one patient rupture of the liver and four fractured ribs.

Safar: You certainly have to avoid pressing on the chest too low, which may rupture the liver, as well as pressing too high, which may fracture the sternum. The lower half of the sternum is the correct location where to apply pressure.

Safar: I now want to change the subject and ask Dr. MAYER to give us her views on the use of *external cardiac compression* in the treatment of *stillborn infants.*

Mayer: Resuscitation of the newborn is different from resuscitation later in life. The newborn lung did not experience regular breathing. The newborn has no acquired heart disease. For the newborn's heart to go into arrest, a long period of asphyxia is required. Prolonged asphyxia inevitably produces irreversible brain damage. Artificial circulation can be easily established in the newborn by external cardiac compression — without instruments — with bare hands. The decision to re-animate such a baby with possible brain damage or to leave it alone has become a problem for the conscience, or the philosophy or the optimism of the resuscitator. I suppose we all feel good playing God and making a stillborn baby live. I think, however, we must keep in mind what a decerebrated child means to himself, to the parents, the siblings, the nurses and the community. Respiratory resuscitation is an entirely different matter. Here again, the newer technique of mouth-to-mouth insufflation has caused a revolution. Rarely, tracheal intubation is necessary any longer if the baby's anatomy is normal. Time is saved and hypoxic brain damage is minimized. The controversy about the value of oxygen administration into the stomach has become academic.

Safar: How would you perform cardiac compression in stillborns?

Mayer: With 2 fingers, about 120 compressions per minute.

Safar: Do you think the trachea should be intubated whenever cardiac compression is used in newborns?

Mayer: No, I do not think tracheal intubation is necessary. It is much faster to go ahead without tracheal intubation.

Zindler: Dr. MAYER, do you give 100% oxygen by mask instead of exhaled air?

Mayer: If you have it, yes.

Safar: We feel differently about the use of the tracheal tube in newborn resuscitation. Since high inflation pressures are usually required to inflate the uninflated or poorly inflated lungs of the newborn, gastric distension is common, unless a tracheal tube is used. We recommend only brief attempts at reoxygenating by bag-mask or mouth-to-mouth. If this does not ventilate adequately within seconds, we intubate the trachea and perform mouth-to-tracheal tube "puffing" or bag-oxygen inflation via tracheal tube.

Is there any evidence that a stillborn can be salvaged with an intact brain after anoxic cardiac arrest had occurred? In other words, is there any evidence that a newborn's normal heart can stop for reasons other than anoxia, before anoxia had damaged the brain permanently?

Members of the Panel: No comments.

Safar: This is a serious question Dr. MAYER raises. A salvaged newborn may survive with brain damage which you may not recognize at the time of resuscitation and for several years thereafter, until you find out that the child is a cerebral cripple.

Zindler: Do you believe that all newborns whose hearts have stopped have already suffered irreversible cerebral damage?

Mayer: Yes, I do. When talking about the child with a normal heart. It is very difficult to stop the normal newborn's heart. I know of a baby with numerous abnormalities whose heart was beating in the presence of complete airway obstruction for several hours.

Safar: MOYA of New York reported on one stillborn infant successfully revived by external cardiac compressions. The baby is well after several months and so far had developed normally with no demonstrable neurologic damage [52]. The end results following the use of external cardiac compression in newborn resuscitation are not known at this time, because it is too early for long-term follow-up examinations. There were 16 babies, resuscitated successfully with the open cardiac massage technique, reported by SUTHERLAND and EPPLE [53]. Most of the babies who survived in this series had some neurologic deficit.

Zindler: I know of the report of one successful cardiac massage by EPPLE and SUTHERLAND [53]. Dr. EPPLE reported later on this baby and a second one [54] and wrote in a letter to me that the first baby had 2 years and 7 months later a slight intentional tremor of the hands and a slight ataxia in walking. His psychic development was undisturbed. The second had two years later, no demonstrable lesions.

The conclusion probably is that one should not try to resuscitate the heart of a newborn once the heart has definitely stopped.

Mayer: Yes, I agree with you. This is a matter of your conscience.

Safar: I also agree in principle. External cardiac compression, however, may have a place for assisted circulation in the pulseless, hypoxic newborn who still has an audible heartbeat.

Mayer: I know of several children 8 or 10 years of age who survived newborn resuscitation but are at the mental level of an infant.

Safar: I think we should give much thought to this problem since one may get into the same difficulty one got into when oxygen was introduced first into the care of premature newborns. This resulted in thousands of blind babies before it was recognized that the high oxygen tensions caused the retrolental fibroplasia. We may start a similar "epidemic" with the introduction of cardiac resuscitation in stillborns.

This much about newborn resuscitation. Let us change the subject.

Safar: What is your experience with *machines* for external cardiac compression?

Negovsky: We have no experience with machines for external cardiac compression.

Lawin: No experience.

Zindler: No experience.

Mayer: No experience.

Harris: Dr. SAFAR and I had experience with the use of the Beck-Rand external cardiac compression machine in the laboratory. This machine provided compressions with constant force and rate in over 60 dog experiments in which supportive maneuvers during external cardiac compression were tested. Artificial arterial pressures and flows were slightly higher during manual sternal compressions, but less variable when the machine was used.

Our experience with this machine in patients, is limited to one case, since external cardiac compression was usually required for only limited periods. We were afraid that in patients applying the machine would cause unnecessary interruptions of the manual compressions and would be too cumbersome at the already overcrowded resuscitation scene. We hope that heart massage machines will never distract from the greatest advantage of external cardiac compression, namely, simplicity, immediate availability and no need for equipment. In ambulance cars, for prolonged sternal compressions during transportation, such machines may prove to be of value. The synchronized mechanical respirators of heart massage machines should only be used in patients whose tracheas are intubated. In the non-intubated patient, one operator must hold the head tilted backward and the mask firmly to the face; he then can ventilate by a Ruben bag or with exhaled air.

These methods enable him to recognize airway obstruction more readily than the use of the machine.

Any other comments?

Israel (Syracuse, New York): Following open heart surgery, would you use closed chest cardiac massage after the chest has been closed or would you open the chest if there is cardiac arrest?

Safar: The Johns Hopkins group has an active cardiac surgical service and is always using the closed technique after the chest is closed following heart surgery — unless there is suspicion of hemorrhage or other intrathoracic complications.

Zindler: The main problem here is that in most cases you are not able to correct the cause of the cardiac arrest, namely, cardiac failure.

If you have a chance to improve the situation by cardiac resuscitation, it is my opinion that you should open the chest because I am convinced that you get a much better circulation by direct compression of these often very large and flabby hearts. With the open method, you can evaluate better the status of the heart and can give easier intra-cardiac injections and also may recognize the presence and the extent of unsuspected or under-estimated hemorrhage. If you have a chance at all, the conditions are much better with opening the chest.

D. Drugs

Safar: Now I would like to change the subject to the use of epinephrine and other drugs. Dr. HARRIS, would you give epinephrine before ventricular fibrillation or standstill has been proven by electrocardiogram?

Harris: My statements are based on dog work and on clinical impressions in humans. Epinephrine should be given as soon as somebody is available to give it, while external cardiac compression is being carried out.

Safar: Do you have evidence that it can do harm if there is fibrillation when you give the epinephrine?

Harris: I have absolutely no evidence that it can do harm. I have some evidence that it helps to defibrillate the heart, as it increases the strength of fibrillation. The stronger the fibrillations are, the easier it is to defibrillate. In addition, the heart comes back with stronger contractions and a better output following the use of epinephrine. If the heart is in standstill, the epinephrine is likely to re-start the heart during massage. If it is in fibrillation, external defibrillation seems easier.

Zindler: How do you diagnose fibrillation?

Harris: You certainly have to wait until the resuscitation cart with the electrocardiograph and defibrillator had arrived at the scene.

Zindler: How would you give the epinephrine?

Harris: We have given it intravenously, based on the fact that the cardiac massage moves blood fairly rapidly. Epinephrine given into the femoral vein of the dog produces an increased artificial blood pressure during the massage within 15 seconds, indicating a fairly rapid circulation into the coronaries.

Safar: Is there also an increase in artificial blood flow during external cardiac compression when epinephrine is given?

Harris: Epinephrine 0.25—1.0 mg. given intravenously during artificial circulation in dogs increased the artificial blood pressure from an average of 80 to 115 mm. Hg; but it had inconsistent effect on the carotid blood flow. Only in a few dogs was the carotid blood flow slightly increased for a short period of time. In most dogs, there was no increase in artificial blood flow.

After defibrillation, however, if we have given epinephrine before, both spontaneous pressure and flow were greatly increased. Therefore, artificial flow was not increased but the spontaneous flow after defibrillation when epinephrine was used was increased.

Safar: The doses used in dogs do not apply to man.

Zindler: Is there any evidence that in asystole epinephrine may cause ventricular fibrillation in man?

Safar: This fear has been stated by ZOLL of Boston, particularly in regard to patients with very diseased hearts. The Johns Hopkins group, however, feels — as we do — that epinephrine should be given as soon as you see that the patient is in cardiac arrest and following the start of cardiac compressions.

Kern: Is there a difference in your opinion between the effect of epinephrine and nor-epinephrine?

Harris: In the dog, both give an excellent rise in artificial pressure during the massage but no rise in flow. After defibrillation, both give a rise in pressure and flow as long as the drug is being given.

Safar: Would you please comment on intracardiac injection?

Harris: Usually, intracardiac injection is not necessary. We give intravenous injection first to avoid interrupting the cardiac compressions, and to prevent possible trauma to the coronary arteries or the lungs with pneumothorax. If intravenous injection is not successful, we use intracardiac injection.

Safar: If intracardiac injection is necessary, it may be safer to inject with a long needle through the costo-xyphoid angle and the diaphragm since this avoids the pleura.

Kern: Intracardiac injection may or may not be effective. In a few instances, I have seen a most impressive improvement after intracardiac injection of both epinephrine and nor-epinephrine in the non-fibrillating heart. Weak and ineffective contractions may be transformed into strong ones and allow shortly afterwards discontinuance of the massage.

Zindler: I am in favor of the intracardiac injection, if it is correctly performed (not into the cardiac muscle or the septum), because it usually requires less time and is more rapidly effective than the intravenous injection.

In patients after circulatory by-pass, we observed that it takes a long time, usually 2 minutes after the intravenous injection of 0.2—2 ml. of 1 : 10,000 epinephrine, until the arterial pressure began to rise, whereas a much smaller dose was more rapidly effective when injected into the heart.

Safar: In actual resuscitations, we inject 1 mg. of epinephrine intravenously immediately after the start of massage. Repeated injections of larger doses were sometimes necessary. We have used a total of 2—4 mg. in asystole without causing fibrillation.

Keszler: Results at our Institute seem to prove that nor-epinephrine is more effective than epinephrine in dogs with cardiac arrest if the drug is applied by intracardiac injection. Our clinical experience supports this view [55]. These and other drugs were, of course, used only in conjunction with massage and/or defibrillation.

Holmdahl: With the discussion of epinephrine we should not forget to discuss the question of acidosis. The sensitivity of the adrenergic receptors is greatly depressed in acidosis. You must increase the dose of epinephrine tremendously in very acidotic patients. I like to quote a case in which we could not restore the heart beat until we had given 10 mg. of epinephrine into the left ventricle. In the acidotic heart you must know that you may have to use enormous doses of epinephrine.

Harris: Was this during circulatory by-pass?

Holmdahl: Yes, immediately after circulatory by-pass in a case of aortic valvular replacement.

Harris: This is different than in brief periods of heart-lung resuscitation. We observed in dogs after 20 minutes of external cardiac compression arterial pH values of 7.0—7.1. With this degree of acidosis epinephrine 0.25—0.5 mg. given intravenously always caused a pronounced pressure effect.

Safar: I would like to ask Dr. HOLMDAHL or Dr. NAHAS whether we should have THAM, bicarbonate, or lactate on our resuscitation carts and when we should inject the alkalinizing substance into the patient's vein.

Nahas: Marked acidosis develops following shock or cardiac arrest. A 60 kg. adult normally produces 200 ml. of CO_2 per minute which corresponds to 10 meq. of titratable acid. One could, therefore, assume that at least this amount of titratable acid accumulates in the body during each minute of circulatory arrest. Furthermore, extensive experimental work has indicated that acidosis will decrease markedly the pressor activity of the catecholamines and also lower the fibrillation threshold of the heart. Conversely, defibrillation of the heart is much more readily obtained when a normal pH prevails [56]. For all these reasons I believe that alkalinizing agents should be administered systematically in the treatment of cardiac arrest. KOUWENHOVEN recommends the early intravenous administration of a solution of $NaHCO_3$ containing 44 meq. which is available in a standard preparation in the emergency ward of every hospital in the United States. This solution is hypertonic. THAM [tris (hydroxymethyl) aminomethane] has not been systematically used clinically in acute cardiac arrest, because this compound has not yet been released for general clinical use [57]. However, it has been used in the treatment of cardiac arrest or fibrillation occurring during open-heart surgery. Dr. R. G. THOMPSON, Department of Surgery, University of Chicago; Dr. R. GROSS, Department of Surgery, Harvard University; and Dr. J. R. MALM, Department of Surgery at Columbia University have all reported instances of cardiac arrest with severe acidosis successfully treated with THAM. The initial dose administered was 1 meq./kg. (120 mg./kg.) of a 0.3 molar solution (isotonic). THAM is a more effective titrating agent than bicarbonate and, in addition, is an intra-cellular buffer. It also acts as an osmotic diuretic and maintains kidney function during surgery and cardiac by-pass, a property which bicarbonate does not have. Anyway, I believe that the treatment of cardiac arrest should include the administration of an alkalinizing agent, either bicarbonate or THAM, to correct the underlying acidosis.

Safar: Can you give too much THAM?

Nahas: One could. However, as much as 1 gm./kg. has been administered during cardiac by-pass, without any ill effect. The dose recommended in the treatment of cardiac arrest (120 mg./kg.) is far below the toxic doses.

THAM depresses ventilation, probably by direct action on the chemosensitive cells of the respiratory center. Therefore, its admistration, when mechanical ventilation is not available, may be hazardous. Large amounts of THAM have also caused hypoglycemia. Subcutaneous infiltration is very irritating as it is accompanied by sloughing of the skin.

Safar: What about sodium lactate?

Nahas: Sodium lactate (40 to 50 ml. of a 1 molar solution) has been used by some investigators (S. BELLET) in the treatment of cardiac arrest. Such a solution may be beneficial because of its high Na content, but not because of its buffering activity. Indeed, sodium lactate is not an effective buffering agent and will not correct the severe acute acidosis associated with cardiac arrest.

Safar: Because of the work Dr. NAHAS has quoted, we are routinely injecting sodium bicarbonate (approximately 44 meq. in 50 ml.) following every 5 minutes of arrest during cardiac resuscitation efforts. Even if spontaneous circulation was restored promptly but there was evidence of poor cardiac output, it would seem rational, at least empirically, to give sodium bicarbonate to combat the metabolic acidosis of inadequate perfusion.

E. Electrocardiography and defibrillation

Safar: Now I would like to ask Dr. NEGOVSKY to comment on defibrillators. The Russians seem to have more experience with direct current defibrillators of the capacitor type, while we have been using primarily the alternating current defibrillators [58]. The voltages presently used most commonly in the U.S.A. are those which produce a current through the heart of over 1 ampere. Such high currents are necessary for defibrillation. Lower currents may cause fibrillation [59]. To obtain such defibrillating currents in adults, between 450 and 1,000 volts AC are used for external defibrillation and between 110 and 220 AC are applied directly to the heart [60]. In both instances, alternating current of 50 to 60 cycles per second is used, with shocks of 0.1—0.25 seconds duration each.

The main advantage of the capacitor discharge DC defibrillator over the AC defibrillator seems to be the fact that the DC defibrillator can be charged from a battery and thus may be portable and not dependent on wall current. Is there any other advantage to the DC defibrillator?

Negovsky: The additional advantages of the capacitor discharge DC defibrillator (i. e. impulse defibrillator) are as follows:

(1.) The shorter period of the shock, which excludes the possibility of additional damage to the cardiac muscle.

(2.) The relative safety for the patient and for the operator.

The basic principle of the electric defibrillation is the achievement of the simultaneous stimulation of all myocardial fibrils produced by a strong electric irritation. Our experiments led us to the conclusion that most effective for this purpose would be the single electric impulse of about 0.01 seconds, the "useful" time for the stimulation of the heart.

The studies made in our laboratory [61] have shown that the current threshold is practically identical whether you use the single impulse (DC discharge) or the more durable stimulation by alternating current (0.2 seconds, i. e. 10 cycles of a 50 cycle/second AC current).

The difference in tension (voltage) is of purely technical nature. During the defibrillation with the aid of an impulse apparatus (capacitor discharge DC defibrillator) the value of the tension on the condenser is three times higher than the tension delivered to the subject. During the defibrillation with an AC defibrillator, the value of the effective tension is a third of the entire amplitude of the tension of both (AC) current phases. Thus, when one compares the value of the tension on both types of defibrillators one must take into account a correction factor of approximately 9.

For *internal* (direct) *defibrillation,* the condenser of the DC defibrillator is charged with 1,500—1,800 volts; when discharged, the current passing from the condenser through the heart corresponds to the one achieved by AC 165—200 volts. For *external defibrillation,* the condenser is charged with 4,000—4,500 volts, which delivers a current through the patient corresponding to the one achieved by AC 440—500 volts.

Safar: It requires 10 to 15 seconds for the capacitor of a DC defibrillator to re-charge. A rapid sequence of shocks, therefore, is not possible. Could the ability to produce serial shocks with the AC defibrillator be an advantage?

Zindler: Yes, sometimes one shock is not sufficient and several shocks have to be used in series.

Negovsky: According to our observations, the phenomenon of the drop of the current threshold by 25—30% when defibrillation is attempted with "iterative irritations" (rapid sequence of shocks, serial shocks), occurs not only with the DC defibrillator but also when AC current is used.

Safar: Who has experience with a DC capacitor discharge defibrillator besides Dr. Negovsky?

Keszler: At our Institute, Dr. Peleska has been working on the problem of DC defibrillation since 1954 [62, 63]. The stimulus for this work came from the publications of Gurvich of Negovsky's

Institute. The first result was the serial production of a DC defibrillator which has proven its value in a considerable number of cases since 1958. On the basis of the statistical analysis of a very considerable amount of experimental work, Dr. PELESKA arrived at the following conclusions:

The electrical current necessary for defibrillation is capable of damaging the heart muscle to a greater or lesser extent. Therefore, it is necessary to choose the parameters which combine maximal efficiency with the least possible damage to the myocardium. Defibrillation requires an impulse of a certain energy (expressed in Joules). In condenser discharges, this energy depends on the relationship between voltage and the size of the condenser. Thus, we may get an impulse of high voltage and short duration or one of low voltage and long duration, both representing the same amount of energy. On evalution of the experimental results, PELESKA found that the optimal duration for DC defibrillation is 10 to 15 milliseconds. Prolonging the impulse beyond this time does not permit lowering of the threshold voltage. The necessary voltage of the impulse is 500—600 volts on the electrodes. The current amounts to 13—20 amperes (also measured on the electrodes). These parameters prove optimal for the DC closed chest defibrillation.

Professor NEGOVSKY mentions 3,500—4,500 volts, but he was obviously speaking of the voltage measured on the condensers, which is higher because the defibrillators used in the Soviet Union also include an inductance choke which lowers the voltage and prolongs the duration of the impulse measured on the electrodes.

For direct (internal, open chest) defibrillation, we use one-third to one-half of the voltage used for indirect (external, closed chest) defibrillation. From the point of view of the energy used, this is only $1/4$ to $1/9$ of the amount necessary for closed chest defibrillation. The necessary voltage depends also on the size of the heart and on the size of the electrodes which should always be as large as necessary to cover the whole heart. The most important results of PELESKA's work are available in two English papers [62, 63].

Safar: When external cardiac compressions have been carried out for several minutes and no spontaneous pulse has returned, should external defibrillating shocks be applied empirically in the absence of an electrocardiograph?

Kern: I have no experience with external defibrillation.

Zindler: I have no practical experience, but I believe that this is advisable especially if the chest cannot be opened and if an electrocardiograph is not available. It is possible that the mechanical stimulation of the hypoxic and acidotic heart by external compressions may cause ventricular fibrillation. If the heart is not fibrillating, no real harm will be done.

Mayer: We would probably perform a thoracotomy within a few minutes. We have no experience with defibrillating shocks in weakly beating hearts or in asystole.

Negovsky: The relative safety and harmlessness of the single electrical impulse (capacitor discharge) allows to recommend this technique in cases when the cardiac activity cannot be restored with the aid of prolonged closed chest massage and the diagnosis of ventricular fibrillation is presumed but not proven. Experiments testing the effect on normal heart action of defibrillatory impulses have shown the absence of apparent disturbances of heart action if the value of the discharge tension is limited by the threshold value.

Safar: What happens if an external defibrillating shock is applied when the heart is in standstill or beating feebly?

Zindler: I do not believe that this will do any harm, besides possibly a local effect. If the current going through the heart is strong enough, and the heart is in standstill, it causes a good contraction of the heart. In a feebly beating heart the same will happen and often it will continue to beat a little stronger than before for 3 to 8 beats. In auricular flutter with tachycardia, the heart may revert to sinus rhythm. This should be tried only if electrocardiographic control is present.

Safar: LOWN and associates recently confirmed the observations made by Dr. NEGOVSKY's group and Dr. PELESKA, namely, that DC countershock in dogs is less injurious to the myocardium than AC and less likely to produce ventricular fibrillation in the normal animal [64]. LOWN recommends an external DC countershock of 2.5 milliseconds duration and 150—200 watt seconds energy.

KOUWENHOVEN showed that currents of less than 0.5 amp. AC, as measured through the dog's heart, produce ventricular fibrillation. Currents of over 1 amp. stop ventricular fibrillation. When applied to the non-fibrillating heart, the high current causes a strong contraction which is followed by escape and spontaneous contractions. The current achieved by a 500 volt 0.25 second AC shock applied through the chest wall of an adult, delivers over 1.5 amp. through the heart since the resistance of the thorax is between 67 and 90 ohms [60].

Poor skin contact or incorrect placement of the electrodes with external countershock may cause fibrillation in a normal heart. The correct placement of the electrodes is one over the suprasternal notch and the other over the apex of the heart. Application of an internal defibrillator shock (110 volts) through the entire chest wall may cause fibrillation.

Safar: Should defibrillators be used in ambulances by para-medical personnel? If yes, should ambulance personnel also learn how to obtain and interpret an electrocardiogram?

Kern: Definitely not.

Zindler: No.

Mayer: No, but a defibrillator and electrocardiograph should be brought to the scene of the accident for use by a physician, rather than bringing the patient to the hospital.

Poulsen: In Denmark, I think that the use of defibrillators in ambulances by para-medical personnel is not relevant because distances to hospitals are moderate. An ambulance will usually be able to reach a well-equipped hospital within 20 minutes, and during the transport ventilation and circulation may be assisted satisfactorily by well-trained ambulance men.

In several cities, an ambulance service has been established in which trained anesthesiologists participate in rescue actions. These physicians will arrive at the scene of the accident within minutes, and in such cases defibrillators and portable electrocardiographs may form an integral part of the equipment.

Harris: I doubt if para-medical personnel could be trained to use an electrocardiograph; in spite of this, the answer to successful resuscitation (particularly in heart attacks and electro-shock victims) may lie in empirical defibrillation as soon as possible.

Safar: External defibrillators in the hands of lay personnel may be justified for especially trained First Aid personnel like those in the electric industry. In general, it seems unwise to put such highly specialized equipment into the hands of para-medical personnel, since, for instance, incorrect application of the electrodes may cause fibrillation in a normal beating heart.

Safar: Does *exsanguinating hemorrhage* in man lead to death in ventricular fibrillation or in asystole?

Negovsky: We have not done electrocardiographic studies in man. The experiments with exsanguinating hemorrhage in dogs have shown that in 5—6 minutes of clinical death 10⁰/₀ stopped in ventricular fibrillation and 90⁰/₀ in asystole.

Zindler: In most patients with exsanguination I saw asystole.

Kern: When the chest was opened in such cases I have seen either ventricular fibrillation or asystole.

Mayer: I have seen asystole with exsanguinating hemorrhage.

Lawin: Cardiac arrests which begin with tachycardia end with ventricular fibrillation. In dogs we have always seen ventricular fibrillation in exsanguinating hemorrhage; also in two men after accidents and in one patient after an operation.

Safar: I have seen several patients exsanguinate while heart action could be observed. As far as I remember, all these hearts stopped in asystole; during resuscitative efforts, however, recurrent episodes of ventricular fibrillation were sometimes observed.

Safar: Is an *external pacemaker* useful for emergency resuscitation of patients who do not have heart block (Stokes Adams Syndrome)?

Negovsky: Yes, it is.

Mayer: I do not think so.

Lawin: No.

Zindler: Definitely not. When we tried a pacemaker applied directly to the heart in patients and in dogs with cardiac arrest, the arterial pressure was always much less than with direct cardiac compressions.

Safar: Dr. ZOLL of Boston feels that the external pacemaker has a place when asystole persists in spite of external compression and the use of epinephrine [*51 b*]. Such cases are rare and may also respond to the mechanical stimulation of the heart by external compressions or pounding of the precordial area. In general, the use of the pacemaker should not be considered a first step in the treatment of cardiac arrest. The exception is the heart block patient who is being monitored, so the pacemaker can take over within seconds of asystole. The hypoxic heart will not contract with pacemaker stimulation, while the oxygenated heart without conduction block usually beats spontaneously.

F. Fluids

Intra-arterial versus intra-venous transfusion

Safar: Before talking about fluid replacement per se, we should discuss the patient with impending cardiac arrest from massive exsanguinating hemorrhage. Experimental work was done in the United States several years ago suggesting that the arterial route of transfusion should be abandoned as it offered no advantage over the intra-venous route [*65*]. Dr. NEGOVSKY has experimental evidence to the contrary. What is the advantage of intra-arterial over intra-venous transfusion in exsanguinating hemorrhage in animals and man?

Negovsky: Time does not permit a detailed discussion of my experiences with intra-arterial transfusion. My experiences are as follows. If the blood pressure is 60 — or below 60, a transfusion of 400 ml. of blood is given intravenously. If after intravenous transfusion of 400 ml. of blood, the arterial pressure does not rise and the venous pressure is rising, we consider this an indication for intra-arterial transfusion [58].

Safar: Is this in dogs or man?

Negovsky: In man and dogs. If the heart is already badly damaged, it is not good enough to try to maintain a blood pressure by massive intravenous transfusion. The intravenous transfusion may actually stop the heart if the heart is already damaged from the oligemic hypotension. Massive intravenous transfusion cannot be tolerated by the heart and the cardiac output will not be increased. In contrast, if the same amount of blood is put into the artery, the output will increase.

Safar: Dr. NEGOVSKY, how do you oxygenate the blood which you pump into the artery?

Negovsky: For 200 ml. of blood, we give 1 ml. of 3% hydrogen peroxide.

Safar: How much oxygen does this give?

Harris: 10 ml. of oxygen in 200 ml. of blood.

Safar: Dr. NEGOVSKY, do you also bubble oxygen through the blood before you pump it into the artery?

Negovsky: Yes, we bubble oxygen through the blood.

Safar: Is there any difference between pulsatile and non-pulsatile infusion? You mentioned in your papers pulsatile infusion.

Negovsky: It does not make any difference.

Safar: There is not time to ask Dr. NEGOVSKY to present his experiments with arterial transfusion. His comments, however, may stimulate us to investigate this question and read about his extensive work on this subject. Most of the work of others was not done with massive exsanguinating hemorrhage, but rather with oligemic hypotension in more or less prolonged shock states.

Harris: In our experiments with dogs in ventricular fibrillation, intra-arterial plasma expanders proved superior to intravenous plasma expanders in equal amounts by raising the carotid blood flow during massage more effectively.

Zindler: Dr. NEGOVSKY, how much blood would you give intra-arterially in 1 minute?

Negovsky: The intra-arterial route is indicated when one has as a goal, the rapid compensation of blood-loss and the restoration of cardiac activity after clinical death, caused by rapid and massive hemorrhage. The rate of the infusion should be 50—60 ml./kg./minute.

Whenever you give blood intra-arterially in order to provoke the reflex stimulation of the circulatory function, as soon as the state of severe traumatic shock (namely, the marked hypotension after blood loss) had been compensated, the rate of infusion may be slowed to 0.2 ml./kg./minute, or a little more.

Zindler: I then doubt the validity of your indication, to use intra-arterial transfusion, if the pressure is below 60 mm. Hg and does not recover after 400 ml. of intravenous transfusion. For example, if you have in this state a cardiac output of 2 liters per minute and then add 300 ml. of blood intra-arterially, how can this make any difference whether you give it intra-arterially or intra-venously?

Safar: Dr. NEGOVSKY, what is the cardiac output in your experimental preparations when you study intra-arterial transfusion? Were your animals close to cardiac arrest?

Zindler: No, with a blood pressure of 60, there must be some cardiac output. Let us say an estimated 2 liters per minute in man. In this case, you are not talking about cardiac arrest.

Negovsky: During 5—6 minutes of clinical death, there is no circulation in animals and therefore no cardiac output. In the first stages of terminal states, when blood pressure is 60 mm. Hg and below 60, there is still cardiac activity and circulation in the organism. Still, the cardiac output as a rule is one-half of the normal then.

Zindler: Sure, 200 to 300 ml. of blood given intra-arterially can change the picture, but also if you give it intravenously. I cannot see how the adding of 200 ml. into the artery can make any difference.

Negovsky: When the blood pressure has *rapidly* dropped below 60 mm. Hg it does not actually make any difference whether you give the blood intra-arterially or intravenously. But if you begin to treat the terminal stage after long-lasting hypotension (blood pressure below 60 mm. Hg), resulting from the *slow* hemorrhage, the arterial technique is much more effective.

There are different ways to give the blood intra-arterially. When, in spite of having increased the volume of the circulating blood following hemorrhage, the hemodynamics are seriously damaged, we use the prolonged (8 to 10 hours) combined transfusion of blood: the drop-by-drop intravenous infusion, associated with fractional periodic infusion of blood into the artery under high pressure, using small amounts — 100 to 150 ml. in 10 to 15 minutes. With this latter technique of intra-arterial transfusion, the more powerful stimulation of the cardio-vascular system is obtained.

In case the blood lost during hemorrhage has not been replaced, one should begin the treatment with rapid intravenous infusion of blood. If, after the infusion of 400 ml. of blood, the arterial pressure does not rise and the venous pressure is rapidly rising, the rate of the intravenous infusion should be slowed and the blood must be given intra-arterially, in portions of 50, 70 and 100 ml. each, with intervals of several seconds or minutes in between.

After a massive hemorrhage when the blood lost had not been sufficiently replaced, one may give the blood intra-arterially, using larger portions of 200—400 ml. or even 500 ml. at one time. Under conditions of continuing massive hemorrhage the volume of the blood given must be equivalent to the volume lost. Great volumes of blood (1.5, 2, 3 liters) should be given intra-arterially, until complete control of hemorrhage has been achieved. After cessation of hemorrhage, the combined intra-arterial-intra-venous infusion normalizes the hemodynamics much more rapidly, although the amounts of the infused blood are smaller [58, 66—69].

Zindler: Another question concerns emergency resuscitation. I believe, if a patient comes into the accident room via ambulance and has massive blood loss, in most hospitals the intravenous cut-down can be made quickly. An intra-arterial cut-down may take 3 to 5 minutes or longer. During this time, it is better to get blood into the vein regardless of whether you think that the arterial or venous transfusion is theoretically better. This is in an emergency resuscitation when time is vital.

Negovsky: I am not trying to discourage the use of intravenous transfusion. In most cases, intravenous transfusion will be effective and one should begin the treatment with it. But in the agonal state, the intra-arterial transfusion should be done first and followed, if necessary, by intravenous infusion of blood. The arterial cut-down (arteria radialis) may take 30 to 40 seconds in the hands of properly trained personnel.

Safar: How rapidly were your animals bled, Dr. NEGOVSKY?

Negovsky: In 15 to 20 minutes, 60 to 70% of blood was drained.

Safar: Dr. NEGOVSKY, do you add any drugs to the intra-arterially transfused blood? What about epinephrine and glucose? Is there any evidence that epinephrine, when injected with the blood into a peripheral artery, can reach the coronary arteries directly, without circulating first through the systemic and pulmonary capillaries?

Negovsky: If the heart is still beating, epinephrine should not be given (neither intra-arterially nor intravenously), unless the restitution of the blood volume has been made. After cardiac arrest the intra-arterial route should be used.

In experiments with 5 minutes of clinical death, where we have not given epinephrine, we could not obtain restoration of cardiac activity. There were few cases in which the heart had been revived, but that two to three times slower than with epinephrine. When epinephrine was given under the same circumstances, the electro-cardiographic alterations, proving the increased myocardial activity, very rapidly appeared in 2 to 3 seconds after injection. This seems to exclude the possibility of an action of the epinephrine via capillaries and pulmonary circulation, because even with normal circulation this would take 8 to 10 seconds. In terminal stages, the rate of the blood flow is very slow. When the heart is not beating, as on the 5th minute of clinical death (the time when we begin the resuscitation of animals), there is no circulation of the blood at all.

Safar: Dr. WOOLMER, do you have any views on the use of intra-arterial vs. intravenous transfusion in exsanguinating hemorrhage?

Woolmer (Director, Research Department of Anaesthetics, Royal College of Surgeons, London): I came to the conclusion that all the views that intra-arterial transfusion may be superior to intravenous transfusion was experimentally disproven. Practically, I think it does not make a great deal of difference which route you choose.

Safar: Dr. WOOLMER, do you know of any work done with intra-arterial transfusion in animals who were bled to the point of cardiac arrest, other than the observations mentioned by Dr. NEGOVSKY?

Woolmer: No, I do not know of any such work.

Nahas: Rapid intra-arterial transfusion via the femoral artery results in a marked increase in coronary blood flow in exsanguinated dogs. This procedure is only beneficial when fresh heparinized blood is used and will result in an improvement of cardiac function. Indeed, if A.C.D. (acid-citrate-dextrose) bank blood is used instead, which has a pH of 6.6 to 6.8, severe cardiac arrhythmias and cardiac arrest may be observed. Then large amounts of epinephrine (0.5 to 1.0 mg./500 ml. of blood) must be added to the blood in order to restore and maintain adequate cardiovascular function [70].

Keszler: HEJHAL and FIRT have done a considerable amount of work on the problems of intravenous and intra-arterial transfusions in severe hemorrhage. Both are working at our Institute for Clinical and Experimental Surgery in Prague and, therefore, I am intimately acquainted with their results which were published in a book that contains a detailed English summary [71]. Their results were also published in many journals including the Lancet [72]. A brief summary of their findings can be given in six points:

(1.) Overloading and eventual failure of the heart in rapid intravenous transfusion is not due to the speed of the transfusion itself, but to the sodium citrate contained in stored blood [72, Fig. 2, 3].

(2.) Citrate causes considerable vasoconstriction in the pulmonary bed and furthermore has a detrimental effect on the myocardium. These mechanisms cause depression of cardiovascular activity resulting in overloading the right heart and heart failure.

(3.) Blood which does not contain citrate (e. g. heparinized blood) may be given at a speed which is far in excess of what is generally considered safe. In post-hemorrhagic hypotension of 60 mm. Hg in dogs, up to 77 ml./kg./min. may be given [72, Fig. 4].

(4.) If calcium is given intravenously at the same time as citrated blood, the admissible speed of transfusion will be the same as with heparinized blood [72, Fig. 7]. The calcium (gluconate or chloride) has to be given into another vein than the transfusion in order to prevent coagulation.

(5.) The apparent advantage of intra-arterial transfusion is due to the fact that a considerable part of sodium citrate contained in stored blood escapes from the capillaries into the interstitial tissues. Consequently, the amount of citrate that reaches the pulmonary vascular bed and the myocardium is much smaller than in intravenous transfusion. Since, however, only part of the citrate escapes, the results of intra-arterial transfusion of stored blood are worse than the results of intravenous transfusion of heparinized blood, or stored blood plus calcium.

(6.) If blood which contains no citrate is used, it is impossible to prove any difference between the effects of intravenous and intra-arterial transfusion.

Safar: FIRT and HEJHAL [72] did not bleed their dogs to cardiac arrest as Dr. NEGOVSKY did, but rather bled them to an arterial pressure of 60 mm. Hg. They transfused after 30 minutes of hypotension. Also, as far as I know, Dr. NEGOVSKY used heparinized blood. Therefore, the experimental conditions in the work of these two investigators were not comparable.

Would you think that in severe cases of exsanguination we should perform thoracotomy with direct manual systole, since this would facilitate the injection of blood into the aorta? This may be faster than the dissection of a peripheral artery.

Keszler: There is a real difference between intravenous and intra-arterial transfusion only in cardiac arrest, since intra-arterial transfusion in this case may often be successful if carried out in time while intravenous transfusion necessarily fails. In spite of this, we are in favor of thoracotomy combined with rapid intravenous transfusion. Calcium has to be given into another vein at the same time, of course. Thoracotomy can be carried out faster and more easily than intra-arterial transfusion, at least in our experience. In addition, resuscitation of the heart requires heparinized blood since, as PELESKA showed in our Institute, citrated blood is unsuitable for this purpose. Although the ill-effects of citrate can be mitigated to a considerable extent by giving calcium simultaneously, cardiac resuscitation by intra-arterial transfusion seems indicated to us only if a suitable artery is already prepared for this purpose. To transfuse blood into the thoracic aorta is impractical in most cases, according to our experience. There is usually too little space to massage the heart efficiently and retain a needle in the aorta safety at the same time.

Kern: I would like to underline what Dr. ZINDLER und Dr. KESZLER had to say on this question of intra-arterial vs. intravenous transfusion. Intra-arterial transfusion may be of utmost importance in research work, but in clinical anesthesia or in clinical resuscitation, it is much more difficult to get a needle into an artery than into a vein and it is more difficult to obtain heparinized blood than citrated blood.

Safar: Could arterial cut-down not become a routine technique in accident rooms of most large hospitals?

Kern: Even then transfusion would be much easier and much more rapidly performed by the intravenous route.

Safar: Thank you. This was an interesting discussion. It may have aroused some renewed interest in arterial transfusion.

Safar: Now a few questions on *fluids in general*. What type of fluid and how much should be given during cardiopulmonary resuscitation and thereafter.

Kern: Everybody will agree that in case of hemorrhage the fluid to be given is blood. However, opinions may differ if there is no obvious evidence of hemorrhage. In the case of traumatic shock — and this is nowadays the most important group of patients requiring emergency resuscitation — there is little doubt that the main cause of circulatory failure is loss of blood, even in the absence of external bleeding. Resuscitation in traumatic shock may require enormous volumes of blood. Our experience in World War II and the reports from the Korean war show convincingly that to restore a proper circulation in traumatic shock, much more blood may be needed than what actually has been lost by the patient.

I think we must stress this point again and again, because those who do not have extensive experience with the treatment of traumatic shock, do not know that a patient may need 15, 20 or even more pints of blood.

I have never seen a shocked patient die from overtransfusion, but I wonder whether in some cases which were called "irreversible traumatic shock", the patient did not die from undertransfusion.

Hypotension from heart failure due to myocardial disease or myocardial infarction is believed to be a definite contra-indication for transfusion. I have little experience with such cases and no definite opinion, but it would be worth while investigating this point again. Tissue anoxia leads so quickly to capillary dilatation and pooling of blood, that even in these cases the filling of the vascular bed might be helpful.

In case of prolonged circulatory failure, I am in favor of blood transfusion in almost every instance. But what shall we do if there is no blood immediately available?

As a temporary measure, plasma expanders may be very useful; we must change to blood as quickly as possible. In my opinion, electrolyte solutions or hypertonic glucose with insulin — as advocated by several French physicians (LABORIT, MICHON, and LARCAN) are of little or no help. These solutions may prove useful for long-term resuscitation, but their usefulness for emergency resuscitation is questionable.

Zindler: In the resuscitation of a patient with hemorrhage it is a common error not to give enough blood. Tremendous amounts may be lost directly or indirectly from the circulating blood volume. It is important in massive transfusions to combat the effect of the lack of free calcium ions and the acidosis. The latter depends on the age of the bank blood. For each pint of blood, we give 5 ml. of calcium 10% and 2 ml. of sodium bicarbonate 6%.

In proven hemorrhage one should give blood until the blood pressure starts to rise or the central venous pressure rises above 20 cm. of water and — in practice — until you see a definite filling of the neck veins.

Safar: Doses anyone in the audience or the panel know how much blood we can return to the circulation by raising the legs? This is the field method of "autotransfusion" recommended to "prime the pump".

Negovsky: About one fifth of the blood volume can be mobilized by raising the legs in man.

Poulsen: Dr. SILBER of Karelia (USSR) conducted experiments on that. He presented his results at this meeting two days ago. By raising the legs of anesthetized adult subjects he succeeded in increasing the volume of the circulating blood by 500—1000 ml.

Safar: Should we give fluids during cardiopulmonary resuscitation even if the cardiac arrest was not associated with blood loss?

Harris: Experimentally in dogs, we found that this was beneficial. Fluids like dextran, given during external cardiac compression, either intravenously or intra-arterially, always increased the carotid flow.

In contrast, giving epinephrine without fluids did not increase the flow, although it increased the pressure.

Safar: Recently, many experts have added important knowledge to the treatment of shock. For instance, the use of low molecular weight dextran seems to be successful in "unplugging" the capillary circulation in the stasis which accompanies circulatory failure. This and other work was discussed in an international symposium on shock [73].

G. Gauging

Evaluation of salvability

Safar: There was no time during the symposium to discuss the following questions: (a.) When should resuscitation *not* be started; (b.) What are the prognostic signs during resuscitation for assessing ultimate survival of an intact mind and body; (c.) When should further resuscitative efforts be abandoned; and (d.) Who shall make the decision?

These are important questions, which cannot be answered by merely analyzing biological scientific facts of salvability. These questions require, in addition, a philosophic appraisal of what is the "quality and quantity of life" [74], what do we consider "dying with dignity", and what is considered ordinary and extraordinary treatment in any given community. In patients in the terminal stages of incurable disease many physicians withhold supportive therapy, such as antibiotics, fluid therapy, tracheotomy, oxygen and artificial ventilation, — as such therapy would prolong the agony and suffering by prolonging biological life. Although this approach has been customary until recently, the availability of modern resuscitation techniques often creates a dilemma for the patient's physician. If resuscitation specialists should agree that biological life without hope for recovery of the mind should not be propagated, physicians must have the courage to discuss this topic frankly. Then, long-term resuscitation following emergency resuscitation should be considered like the supportive measures, which are being used so widely in our decerebrated, chronically ill aged citizens, preventing them from dying with dignity [75].

I have not asked the members of the panel to comment on these questions by correspondence, since only personal discussion could do justice to such a controversial and delicate topic. In our medical student's program in anesthesia and resuscitation at the University of Pittsburgh, these questions are discussed in seminar sessions, which invariably lead to much controversy.

For the sake of completeness of the "ABC" of resuscitation in this published version of our symposium, however, I am taking the liberty of quoting some of my own views [76]:

When Should Resuscitation Efforts be Discontinued?

Although modern resuscitation undoubtedly can save many patients who were considered non-salvable in the past, it has changed the definition of death. Cessation of breathing movements and absence of pulse and heart sounds can no longer be considered signs of death. Death should be defined as "evidence of irreversible cerebral destruction".

When a patient is found in acute respiratory or circulatory distress and he is not known to be in the terminal stages of an incurable disease, he should be considered salvable and treated promptly with a complete resuscitative effort. There is no time for meditation, contemplation and consultation about diagnosis of the underlying disorder or questions of salvability before starting re-oxygenation of the brain. One must act according to a resuscitation plan prepared and learned ahead of time (Table 2).

After the baseline of cerebral oxygenation has been established, the situation should be assessed and unnecessary prolongation of the act of dying avoided, if the underlying disorder appears incompatible with survival or if there is clear-cut evidence that the hypoxic episode had produced irreversible cerebral damage.

Rapid recovery of reflexes is a good prognostic sign, while progressive deterioration of reflexes and continuing unconsciousness are poor prognostic signs. In children, resuscitation efforts should be continued for longer periods of time since complete neurologic and psychologic recovery has been seen even after unconsciousness of over 1 week duration following a hypoxic insult [77]. It is often difficult to predict the degree of cerebral recovery immediately following resuscitation.

Artificial ventilation and circulation should be continued until either effective spontaneous circulation is restored or — if this is unsuccessful — until signs of cerebral deterioration recur. This is the case when the pupils, which had become smaller at first with cardiopulmonary resuscitation, start dilating again and when reflexes and breathing movements, which had initially returned, are again disappearing.

If, after restoration of spontaneous circulation long-term resuscitative efforts have been started because the patient had not regained consciousness promptly, the physician should use common sense and reach an ethical and humane solution of the problem. If cerebral destruction is obvious, the physician should not hesitate to discontinue long-term resuscitative efforts, after consultation with resuscitative specialists and in consideration of the family situation. Phases I and II of resuscitation are not costly. However, long-term resuscitation (Phase III) and survival of a patient with severe brain damage may create an unbearable financial and emotional burden. No hard and fast rules can be established, since professional judgement, philosophies, religion and finances all play a role in this problem.

Although any salvable patient deserves an all-out modern resuscitative effort, the physician should not forget that the dying patient with known incurable disease deserves a peaceful death with dignity.

H. Hypothermia I. Intensive care

Safar: Now a few questions on hypothermia. Dr. KUCHER, when should hypothermia be started following successful restoration of the heart beat?

Kucher: After successful restoration of spontaneous circulation, hypothermia is indicated in my opinion in all cases in which cardiac arrest may have lasted for more than 3 minutes, if spontaneous respirations did not return within 1—2 hours. It proved to be helpful if there was a severe degree of anoxia.

Safar: ROSOMOFF showed that experimental cerebral ischemia produced during the hypothermic state is followed by less brain damage than the same injury produced under normothermia [78]. Even if hypothermia is induced following the ischemic episode, damage is reduced [79]. Following experimental trauma, the "inflammatory" swelling of the brain is less if the body temperature is lowered for 1 hour or more immediately following the trauma [80]. In cardiac arrest cases, the earlier the body temperature was lowered following cessation of circulation, the greater was the apparent protection provided by hypothermia against post-traumatic edema and permanent cerebral damage, both in animals and man [81].

Respiratory alkalosis due to hyperventilation leads to a reduction in cerebral blood flow [82] and intra-cranial blood volume [83]. In contrast, there is an increase in cerebral blood flow and intra-cranial blood volume with hypercarbia. My associates and I, therefore, feel that immediately following an anoxic insult, the oxygen tension should be raised, and the carbon dioxide tension should be lowered slightly by controlled hyperventilation. The venous pressure should be decreased by keeping the mean airway pressure low and by elevating the head. Cerebral edema should be minimized by early cooling.

Mayer: I agree but it is important to avoid shivering.

Safar: Dr. KUCHER, when would you cool the patient, how low and how long?

Kucher: We use 30 degrees rectally for several days with spontaneous breathing. Shivering is controlled with the "lytic cocktail".

Safar: We use 30 degrees esophageal temperature for not more than 4 days. More prolonged hypothermia leads often to pulmonary complications. We stop shivering preferably with the use of muscle relaxants, to avoid depression of the central nervous system. Curare-like drugs can be discontinued at any time in order to permit observation of the state of consciousness. This is not possible with the use of the "lytic cocktail". The use of relaxants certainly makes mechanical controlled hyperventilation mandatory.

With the use of depressant drugs like the "lytic cocktail" and spontaneous respirations, we found it difficult to control shivering and at the same time be certain that hypercarbia is avoided and that convulsions or restlessness will not impair ventilation or circulation. Also, the patient may remain unconscious because of the drugs rather than the anoxic insult.

Negovsky: I agree with what was said. We are using prolonged hypothermia of approximately 30 degrees following cardiac arrest.

Mayer: We have another indication, namely, fever. We should not let the temperature of the patient rise.

Safar: Certainly, one should also use external cooling not only to produce hypothermia but also to prevent hyperthermia.

Zindler: What do you think about putting the ice directly on the head when you start cooling?

Safar: I think there is evidence that you do not get cerebral cooling any faster by local application of cold to the head.

Zindler: No, I meant not only local cooling but the whole body including the head and neck, with the idea to try to apply cold also where you want it, namely, at the brain.

Comment from the Audience: One should consider the speed of cooling by choosing the method properly.

Safar: This is an excellent point, because the beneficial effect of hypothermia following cardiac arrest depends on immediate cooling. Rapid cooling is much easier in the dog. What do we gain if we pack a patient into ice 30 minutes after the cardiac arrest and then it takes another hour to reduce the esophageal temperature to 30 degrees. Should we consider extracorporeal cooling whenever the eye reflexes and airway reflexes are not starting to improve 30 minutes after cessation of circulation and successful restoration of cardiac action? Should we apply ice prophylactically as soon as resuscitation efforts are started? Should we use hypertonic solutions, such as urea, to prevent cerebral edema?

Poulsen: Urea has been used by our neurosurgeons during recent years to reduce the volume of the brain during craniotomy, but cerebral edema has developed post-operatively in several cases. Consequently, urea cannot be recommended in the prevention of cerebral edema after resuscitation.

Safar: Although the volume of brain tissue is decreased by urea at the expense of an increase of intra-cranial blood volume, it was shown that there is rebound brain swelling [84, 85]. For this reason, we dot not use urea following an anoxic insult.

Kern: What about concentrated serum albumin?

Safar: I believe this acts the same way as urea. The hypertonic substance distributes through the body and eventually diffuses into all tissues including the brain cells causing delayed swelling.

What are your indications for prolonged mechanical artificial ventilation following restoration of a spontaneous heartbeat?

Harris: If the patient does not regain consciousness immediately, intermittent positive pressure ventilation should be performed until he regains consciousness.

Poulsen: During the last year or so in my department, we have used respirator treatment after initial resuscitation. We do not attempt to hyperventilate the patients, but we aim at an arterial Po_2 and Pco_2 within normal limits.

Safar: We are using controlled hyperventilation (1) to further reduce brain size or at least prevent cerebral congestion and edema during the recovery phase; (2) to combat the metabolic acidosis which follows cardiac arrest; and (3) to abolish the work of breathing.

Kucher: We are using spontaneous breathing with hibernating drugs to stop shivering. We did not measure Pco_2, but only pH, which remained normal.

Safar: When hypothermia is used with spontaneous breathing, one should monitor arterial pH and Pco_2 and start controlled hyperventilation at the first sign of hypercarbia and/or acidosis.

Zindler: Hyperventilation may not be the best thing for the brain, since it decreases cerebral circulation.

Safar: Would you then be in favor of blood gas monitoring to prevent both hypo- and hyperventilation?

Zindler: Yes. We try to keep the P_{CO_2} between 35 and 40 mm. Hg.

Safar: However, in the absence of blood gas measurements, you have to hyperventilate mildly as a safety factor.

Zindler: Prolonged mechanical ventilation (with or without hypothermia) should only be done when there is hope that no irreversible brain damage has occurred.

Indications are: insufficient spontaneous breathing, respiratory distress, conditions which impair adequate ventilation or perfusion of the lungs, and selected cases of cerebral and pulmonary edema.

Heart failure resistant to digitalis, restoration of a normal acid-base balance or epinephrine infusion, is also considered an indication for respirator ventilation, as this relieves the patient of the increased work of respiration. One can improve the oxygen supply to the tissues by control of the inhaled oxygen concentration and by improving alveolar ventilation and possibly decreasing venous admixture by correcting or preventing atelectasis.

Lawin: If spontaneous respirations are inadequate (arterial P_{CO_2} over 55 mm. Hg) or metabolic acidosis is evident, artificial ventilation should be used.

Negovsky: We use the prolonged mechanical artificial respiration in cases when the spontaneous respiration does not assure adequate gas exchange. Most useful are apparatus based on the regulation of the volume of the insufflated air-mixtures or oxygen. With this aid it is much easier to maintain the constant desirable ventilation.

Kern: When spontaneous breathing is not resumed after about half an hour following restoration of the heart beat, we switch from manual to mechanical ventilation. I must say that the prognosis is usually bad if restoration of spontaneous breathing is delayed.

Safar: Our time is up. I want to thank the panel members and the audience for their contributions and for their patience.

Addendum

Safar: Long-term resuscitation is beyond the scope of this panel. It should be considered part of the duty of anesthesia departments in large hospitals, not only to establish, organize and train an *emergency* resuscitation team [76], but also to provide a *long-term* resuscitation service, best in an Intensive Care Unit [86, 87].

Intensive Care includes: Inhalational therapy, tracheotomy, tracheotomy care, prolonged artificial ventilation, general care of the unconscious patient, monitoring, fluid and electrolyte balance and the circulatory support by drugs.

Table 5. *Cardio-pulmonary*

	Reported by	Institution	Period
(A) In hospital, outside op. rooms and recov. rooms	BECK	Lakeside Hosp. Cleveland	15 yrs. 47/62
	JUDE	Johns Hopkins Hosp. Baltimore	46 mo. 59/62
	SAFAR, WILDER	Baltimore City Hospital	30 mo. 60/62
	SAFAR, HARRIS	Presb.-Univ. Hosp. Pittsburgh	15 mo. 62/63
	POULSEN	Univ. Hosp. Aarhus	18 mo. 61/62
	KESZLER	Surg. Res. Dpt. Prague	15 mo. 61/62
	KERN	Univ. Hosp.s Paris	12 mo. 61/62
	NEGOVSKY	Lab. for Resus. Moscow	12 mo. 62/63
	MAYER	Bellevue Hosp. New York	24 mo. 61/62
	HOLMDAHL, GRÄNGSJÖ	Univ. Hosp. Upsala	24 mo. 61/63
	LAWIN	Univ. Hosp. Hamburg	12 mo. 61/62
	KLASSEN [*88*]	Royal Vict. Hosp. Montreal	18 mo. 61/62
(B) Start of resusc. outside hosp., cont in hosp.	JUDE, WILDER	Baltimore Ambulance S.	36 mo. 60/63
	POULSEN	To Univ. Hosp. Aarhus	18 mo. 61/62
	NEGOVSKY	Lab. for Resus. Moscow	12 mo. 62
	KERN	Univ. Hosp. Paris	12 mo. 61/62
	BECK	Lakeside Hosp. Cleveland	15 yrs. 47/62

* Internal cardiac compression via thoracotomy. All other figures refer to external cardiac compression.

** Number of arrests.

resuscitation attempts outside operating rooms

Cause of arrest	No.pts. resusc. attempted	No.resusc. to spont. cardiac action	No.resusc. to prearrest cardiac and CNS status	No.pts. left hospital
Coron.	(?)*32	?	?	9*
Other	25* 50	?	?	2* 10
Coron.	47	22**	11**	7
Other	98	87**	51**	19
Coron.	over 50	(?)	1	1
Other	over 100	(?)	(?)	4
Coron.	over 50	(?)	6	5
Other	over 50	(?)	(?)	6
Coron.	1	1	0	0
Other	4	3	2	1
Coron.	1	0	0	0
Other	11	9	6	3
Coron.	0	0	0	0
Other	3	2	0	0
Coron.	20	14	4	4
Other	11	4	2	1
Coron.	over 2	2	2	2
Other	over 1	1	1	1
Coron.	9	6	3	3
Other	42	31	13	12
Coron.	0	0	0	0
Other	4	4	3	3
Coron.	46	10	?	4
Other	40	9	?	6
Total	101	12	3	2***
Coron.	14	2	1	0
Other	5	2	2	1
Coron.	3	3	3	3
Total	1	1	1	1
Coron.	?	?	1*	1*
Total approx.	over 821	?	?	111

*** 5 additional patients with questionable arrests "revived" during transportation (personal communication).

Reports
on cardio-pulmonary resuscitation attempts
outside of the operating rooms

Safar: Most Anesthesiologists have first-hand experience with cardiopulmonary resuscitation in the operating rooms and the recovery rooms. Cardiac arrest in these areas in most instances is readily detected and competently treated, as anesthesiologists and surgeons are immediately available. In contrast, cardio-pulmonary resuscitation attempts outside the operating rooms and the recovery rooms have been rare. Following the introduction of mouth-to-mouth ventilation and external cardiac compression, however, cardiac resuscitation attempts on the wards, in the emergency room, and some even outside of hospitals, are increasing in number. The salvage rates in these areas so far, have been low, since many of these patients are suffering from incurable disease and often resuscitation is started too late to permit recovery of the central nervous system. More extensive teaching of the early recognition and treatment of cardio-pulmonary collapse, better organization of resuscitation services and better monitoring and alarm systems, we hope, will increase the salvage rate.

The members of the symposium submitted, by mail, the results they know of with cardio-pulmonary resuscitation attempts outside of the operating rooms and recovery rooms. These reports are summarized in Table 5 (see pages 56/57).

Summary

This symposium was an exchange of views rather than a presentation of original data. The following conclusions concerning the discussion of practical points may be justified:

(1.) The number of deaths, possibly reversible by prompt, modern resuscitation efforts is much greater than usually assumed. Even some of the sudden deaths associated with coronary heart disease are reversible.

(2.) Cardiac arrest is defined as "the clinical picture of cessation of circulation (unconsciousness; pulselessness of large arteries; apnea or changed respiration; and gray color) in a person who is not expected to die at the time".

(3.) A plan of action for the treatment of respiratory and circulatory emergencies was outlined in alphabetic order.

(4.) The most important steps in the management of airway obstruction and apnea are backward tilt of the head and positive pressure inflation attempts through mouth and nose. Tracheal intubation and tracheotomy should be preceded by re-oxygenation attempts through mouth and nose. The place of crico-thyroid membrane puncture deserves further evaluation.

(5.) In emergency resuscitation, intermittent positive pressure ventilation with "lung operated" (exhaled air) or hand-operated (bag or bellows-mask) methods is superior to the use of automatic resuscitators.

(6.) For emergency re-oxygenation, high oxygen tensions (if available) are preferable to air. Following prolonged hypoxia (agony) in dogs, NEGOVSKY observed harm from prolonged ventilation with pure oxygen. No convincing evidence was presented that high alveolar oxygen tensions (below one atmosphere) are contraindicated in emergency and long-term artificial ventilation in man.

(7.) Emergency artificial circulation is started most rapidly by external cardiac compressions (rhythmic sternal pressure). This must be accompanied by intermittent positive pressure ventilation. One of several satisfactory ratios is 2—3 inflations/15 sternal compressions. Interposing lung inflations is easier when the trachea is intubated.

(8.) Internal cardiac compressions via thoracotomy may be mechanically more effective in some cases, should be reserved for operating room emergencies, and should be preceded by external cardiac resuscitation attempts, unless the thorax is already open.

(9.) In newborn infants without audible heartbeat, it is doubtful whether cardiac resuscitation attempts are justified. Sternal compressions, however, may be indicated to assist feeble cardiac contractions in the newborn.

(10.) In cardiac arrest, clinical experience indicates that epinephrine should be given intravenously or intracardially even before diagnosis and treatment of ventricular fibrillation. The metabolic acidosis accompanying cardiac arrest should always be counteracted by alkalinizing agents.

(11.) External defibrillation is an established procedure. The use of DC capacitor discharge defibrillators offer some advantages over the use of AC countershocks. Empirical countershock by para-medical personnel is not recommended at this time. The use of external pacemakers is not a first step in emergency resuscitation, except for cases of heart block.

(12.) The place of intra-arterial transfusion deserves further studies. In exsanguination and after prolonged agony (irreversible shock), intra-arterial transfusion may be superior to intravenous transfusion. The superiority of heparinized over citrated blood in massive transfusions is more pronounced with the intravenous than with the intra-arterial route.

(13.) "Resuscitology" is changing the definition of death. Decisions when not to start resuscitation and when to abandon resuscitation efforts must be made.

(14.) Whenever recover of reflexes and consciousness are delayed, hypothermia, prolonged mechanical controlled ventilation and intensive medical and nursing care should be started as soon as possible following cerebral hypoxia.

Bibliography

[1] Facts on Killing and Crippling Diseases in U.S.A. The National Health Education Committee, Inc., 135 East 42nd Street, New York, U.S.A., Pgs. 2, 12.
[2] American National Red Cross, Washington, D. C. Accident Facts. Personal communication, Dr. Sam T. Gibson.
[3] SAFAR, P., L. A. AGUTO-ESCARRAGA, and F. CHANG: A study of upper airway obstruction in the unconscious patient. J. appl. Physiol. **14**, 760 (1959).

[4] MORIKAWA, S., P. SAFAR, and J. DeCARLO: Influence of head position upon upper airway patency. Anesthesiology 22, 265 (1961).

[5] CHASE, H. F., M. A. KILMORE, and R. M. TOMASELLO: Effect of respiratory obstruction on brain size and motion. Anesthesiology 23, 142 (1962).

[6] WHITE, J. C., M. VERLOT, B. SELVERSTONE, and H. K. BEECHER: Changes in brain volume during anesthesia: The effects of anoxia and hypercapnia. Arch. Surg. 44, 1 (1942).

[7] International Symposium on Emergency Resuscitation. Acta anaesth. scand. Suppl. IX (1961).

[8] KOUWENHOVEN, W. B., J. R. JUDE, and G. G. KNICKERBOCKER: Closed chest cardiac massage. J. Amer. med. Ass. 173, 1064 (1960).

[9] BECK, C. S.: The fatal heart attack. Personal publication. Western Reserve University, Cleveland, Ohio, 1962, and LEIGHNINGER, D. S.: Personal communication.

[10] JUDE, J. R., W. B. KOUWENHOVEN, and G. G. KNICKERBOCKER: Cardiac arrest. Report of application of external cardiac massage on 118 patients. J. Amer. med. Ass. 178, 1063 (1961).

[11] WILDER, R.: Personal communication.

[12] ADELSON, L., and W. HOFFMAN: Sudden death from coronary artery disease. A statistical study, Cuyahoga County Coroner's Office, Cleveland. J. Amer. med. Ass. 176, 129 (1961).

[13] BECK, C. S., and D. S. LEIGHNINGER: Scientific basis for the surgical treatment of coronary artery disease. J. Amer. med. Ass. 159, 1264 (1955).

[14] PHILLIPS, O. C., and T. M. FRAZIER: The Baltimore Anesthesia Study Committee. Organization and preliminary report. Anesthesiology 18, 33 (1957).

[15] PHILLIPS, O. C., T. M. FRAZIER, T. D. GRAFF, and T. J. DeKORNFELD: The Baltimore Anesthesia Study Committee. J. Amer. med. Ass. 174, 2015 (1960).

[16] DRIPPS, R. D., A. LAMONT, and J. E. ECKENHOFF: The role of anesthesia in surgical mortality. J. Amer. med. Ass. 178, 261 (1961).

[17] BEECHER, H. K., and D. T. TODD: A study of the deaths associated with anesthesia and surgery. Springfield, Ill.: Thomas 1954.

[18] PHILLIPS, O. C., T. M. FRAZIER, and G. H. DAVIS: Factors in obstetric mortality. Amer. J. Obstet. Gynec. (in press).

[19] Münch. med. Wschr. 102/7, 351 (1960).

[20] ROSSEN, R., H. KABAT, and J. P. ANDERSON: Acute arrest of cerebral circulation in man. Arch. Neurol. Psychiat. (Chic.) 50, 510 (1943).

[21] HOLMDAHL, M. H.: Pulmonary uptake of oxygen, acid-base metabolism, and circulation during prolonged apnoea. Acta chir. scand., Suppl. 212 (1956).

[22] ELAM, J. O., E. S. BROWN, and J. D. ELDER JR.: Artificial respiration by mouth-to-mask method. Study of respiratory gas exchange of paralyzed patients ventilated by operator's expired air. New Engl. J. Med. 250, 749 (1954).

[23] SAFAR, P., L. ESCARRAGA, and J. ELAM: A comparison of the mouth-to-mouth and mouth-to-airway methods of artificial respiration with the chest-pressure arm-lift methods. New Engl. J. Med. 258, 671 (1958).

[24] Symposium on Mouth-to Mouth Resuscitation. J. Amer. med. Ass. 167, 317 (1958).

[25] SAFAR, P.: The failure of manual respiration. J. appl. Physiol. **14**, 84 (1959).

[26] SAPOV, I. A.: Role of the Nervous System in Mechanism of Oxygen Toxicity. Dissertation, Leningrad (1962).

[27] SIROTININ, N. N.: Influence of hyper-oxygenation on the living organism. Oxygen therapy and oxygen toxicity. Pgs. 148—163. Kiev: 1952.

[28] BERT, P.: La pression barometrique Recherches de physiologie experimentale. Paris: 1878.

[29] COMROE, J. H., R. D. DRIPPS, P. DUMKE, and M. DEMING: Oxygen toxicity. J. Amer. med. Ass. **128**, 710 (1945).

[30] COMROE, J. H., E. R. BAHNSON, and E. O. COATES: Mental changes occurring in chronically anoxemie patients during oxygen therapy. J. Amer. med. Ass. **143**, 1044 (1950).

[31] GRANDPIERRE, R., C. A. FRANCK, et R. LEMAIRE: L'éxcitabilité du centre respiratoire dans l'action paradoxale de l'oxygène. C. R. Soc. Biol. (Paris) **142**, 1028 (1948).

[32] GRANDPIERRE, R., C. A. FRANCK et R. LEMAIRE: L'action paradoxale de l'oxygène. J. Physiol. (Paris) **421**, 5 (1950).

[33] SMIRENSKAYA, E. M., and N. P. ROMANOVA: Oxygen therapy in the recovery period after clinical death. Byull. éksp. Biol. Med. **9**, 66—71 (1958).

[34] NEGOVSKY, V. A., A. MILHAUD, N. L. GURVICH, and E. S. ZOLOTOKRYLINA: Application of indirect heart massage with sudden ventricular fibrillation. Exp. Surg. Anesth. **5**, 3 (1962).

[35] REDDING, J., R. COZINE, G. VOIGT, and P. SAFAR: Resuscitation from drowning. J. Amer. med. Ass. **178**, 1136 (1961).

[36] FREEMAN, J., and J. F. NUNN: Personal communication, 1961.

[37] Emergency Resuscitation Symposium. Acta anaesth. scand., Suppl. IX (1961), pg. 203.

[38] ROSEN, M., and E. K. HILLARD: The use of suction in clinical medicine. Brit. J. Anaesth. **32/10**, 486 (1960).

[39] SAFAR, P., T. BROWN, W. HOLTEY, and R. WILDER: Ventilation and circulation with closed-chest cardiac massage in man. J. Amer. med. Ass. **176**, 574 (1961).

[40] Emergency Resuscitation Symposium. Acta anaesth. scand., Suppl. IX (1961), pg. 133.

[41] REDDING, J., and R. COZINE: A comparison of open-chest and closed-chest cardiac massage in dogs. Anesthesiology **22**, 280 (1961).

[42] WEALE, F. E., and R. L. ROTHWELL-JACKSON: The efficiency of cardiac massage. Lancet **1962**, 990—992.

[43] DOWNS, T. M.: Carotid sinus as etiological factor in sudden anesthetic death. Ann. Surg. **99**, 974 (1934).

[44] WEISS, S., and J. P. BAKER: Carotid sinus reflex in health and disease; its rule in causation of fainting and convulsions. Medicine (Baltimore) **12**, 297 (1933).

[45] SIGLER, L. H.: Hyperactive cardio-inhibitory carotid sinus reflex; possible aid in diagnosis of coronary disease. Arch. intern. Med. **67**, 177 (1941).

[46] BURSTEIN, C. L., B. J. CILIBERTI, E. CRAWFORD, J. MARIN, L. C. MARK, V. D. B. MAZZIA, and G. WALLACE: Clinical anesthesia conference. N. Y. St. J. Med. **58/16**, 2697 (1958).

[47] DWYER, C. J., P. B. THOMAS, and W. G. STROUT: Cardiac arrest on intubation. Anesth. Analg. Curr. Res. 32, 123 (1953).

[48] KING, R. D., L. C. HARRIS, F. E. GREIFENSTEIN, J. D. ELDER, and R. D. DRIPPS: Reflex circulatory responses to direct laryngoscopy and tracheal intubation performed during general anesthesia. Anesthesiology 12, 556 (1951).

[49] HARRIS, L. C., H. G. KUNKEL, and P. SAFAR: Cardiopulmonary resuscitation. A laboratory evaluation. Anesthesiology 24, 132 (1963).

[50] SAFAR, P., T. BROWN, and W. HOLTEY: Failure of closed chest cardiac massage to produce pulmonary ventilation. Dis. Chest 41, 1 (1962).

[51] —, J. O. ELAM, J. JUDE, R. WILDER, and P. M. ZOLL: Resuscitative principles for sudden cardiopulmonary collapse. Panel discussion. Dis. Chest 43, 34 (1963); (a) pg. 42; (b) pg. 47.

[52] MOYA, F., L. S. JAMES, E. BURNARD, and E. C. HANKS: Closed chest cardiac massage in the newborn. Anesthesiology 22, 644 (1961).

[53] SUTHERLAND, J. M., and H. H. EPPLE: Cardiac massage of still born infants. Obstet. Gynec. Survey 18, 182 (1961).

[54] EPPLE, H. H., and J. M. SUTHERLAND: Heart massage for the resuscitation of the newborn. Münch. med. Wschr. 103, 1267 (1961).

[55] SMETANA, J., et E. RACENBERG: A propos du traitement de l'arrest cardiaque. Agressologie I, 363 (1960).

[56] CLARK, L. C.: The use of amine buffers in cardiovascular surgery. Ann. N. Y. Acad. Sci. 92, 687 (1961).

[57] NAHAS, G. G.: Use of an organic carbon dioxide buffer in vivo. Science 129, 782 (1959).

[58] NEGOVSKY, V. A.: Resuscitation and artificial hypothermia. Consultants Bureau (New York), 1962.

[59] PREVOST, J. L., et F. BATTELLI: La mort par les courants electriques-courants alternatifs a haute tension. J. Physiol. Path. gén. 1, 427 (1899).

[60] KOUWENHOVEN, W. B.: Personal communication. See SAFAR, P.: Questions and answers. Anesth. Analg. Curr. Res. 42, 63 (1963).

[61] GURVICH, N. L.: Fibrillation and defibrillation of the heart. Medgez. (Moscow), 1957.

[62] PELESKA, B.: A High Voltage Defibrillator and the Theory of High Voltage Defibrillation. Proc. Third Intern. Conf. on Med. Electronics. (London), Tunbridge Wells, Kent: C. Baldwin Ltd. 1960.

[63] — Cardiac arrhythmias following condenser discharges and their dependence upon voltage and amount of electric energy. Circulat. Res. (in press).

[64] LOWN, B., J. NEUMAN, R. AMARASINGHAM, and B. V. BERKOVITS: Comparison of alternating current with direct current electroshock across the closed chest. Amer. J. Cardiol. 10, 223 (1962).

[65] MALONEY, J. V., C. M. SMYTHE, J. P. GILMORE, and S. W. HANDFORD: Intra-arterial and intravenous transfusion. Surg. Gynec. Obstet. 97, 529 (1953).

[66] ZOLOTOKRILINA, E. S., N. S. KALGANOVA, N. M. RYBOVA, and T. PAVLOVA: Treatment of hemodynamic disorders in traumatic shock and the terminal state. Ortop. Travm. Protez. 12, 9 (1961) (Russia).

[67] — Influence of prolonged animation on the effectiveness of intravenous and intra-arterial transfusion of blood. Pat. Fiziol. éksp. Ter. I, 5, 68 (1957).

[68] KISELEVA, K. S.: On methods of transferring supercharged arterial blood in the treatment of prolonged hypotension, blood loss and shock. Obstet. Gynec. **2**, 42—43 (1962).

[69] NEGOVSKY, V. A.: Some physiopathologic regularities in the process of dying and resuscitation. Circulation **23**, 452 (1961).

[70] NAHAS, G. G.: The use of 2-amino-2-hydroxymethyl-1,3-propanedial in the correction of addition acidosis and its effect on sympatho-adrenal activity. Ann. N. Y. Acad. Sci. **92**, 596 (1961).

[71] HEJHAL, L., and P. FIRT: Otázky léčeni prudkeho krvaceni. Sborn. lék. Prague (1954).

[72] FIRT, P., and L. HEJHAL: Treatment of severe haemorrhage. Lancet **1957 II**, 1132.

[73] Shock. Pathogenesis and Therapy. An International Symposium. Heidelberg: Springer 1962.

[74] LONG, P. H.: On the quantity and quality of life. The Resident Physician **6/4**, 69; **6/5**, 53; **6/6**, 51 (1960).

[75] AYD, F. J.: The hopeless case. J. Amer. med. Ass. **181**, 1099 (1962).

[76] SAFAR, P.: The physician's role in modern resuscitation. Curr. Dig. (Williams & Wilkins, Baltimore) **30**, 53 (1963).

[77] RAVITCH, M., R. LANE, P. SAFAR, F. STEICHEN, and P. KNOWL. Lightning stroke. Recovery following cardiac massage and prolon ged artificial respiration. New Engl. J. of Med. **264**, 36 (1961).

[78] ROSOMOFF, H. L.: Hypothermia and cerebral vascular lesions: Experimental interruption of the middle cerebral artery dur hypothermia. J. Neurosurg. **13**, 244 (1956).

[79] — Hypothermia and cerebral vascular lesions. II. Experiment cerebral artery interruption followed by induction of hyp Arch. Neurol. Psychiat. (Chic.) **78**, 454 (1957).

[80] —, K. SHULMAN, R. RAYNOR, and W. GRAINGER: Experimer injury and delayed hypothermia. Surg. Gyn. Obstet. **110**,

[81] WILLIAMS JR., G. R., and F. C. SPENCER: The clinical use thermia following cardiac arrest. Ann. Surg. **148**, 462 (19⁵

[82] KETY, S. S., and C. F. SCHMIDT: The effects of active an hyperventialation on cerebral blood flow, cerebral oxygen c p-tion, cardiac output, and blood pressure in young men Invest. **25**, 107 (1946).

[83] ROSOMOFF, H. L.: The distribution of intra-cranial conter witl controlled hyperventilation. Implications for neuroaɪ ɜthesia. Anesthesiology (in press).

[84] — Distribution of intracranial contents after hypertonic urea. J. Neurosurg. **19**, 859 (1962).

[85] LOEHNING, R. W., H. UEYAMA, and I. UEDA: Brain volume studies in animals: Effects of hypercarbia, hypoxia, and intravenous urea. Anesth. Analges. **41**, 529 (1962).

[86] SAFAR, P.: Intensive care unit. Anaesthesia **16**, 275 (1961).

[87] HOLMDAHL, M. H.: The respiratory care unit. Anesthesiology **23**, 559 (1962).

[88] KLASSEN, G. A., C. BROADHURST, and A. L. JOHNSON: Cardiac resuscitation in 86 medical patients using external cardiac massage. Meeting, Canadian Cardiovascular Soc. Nov. 1962.